Pra

MW01290767

"I have been a pastor and pastoral counselor for over forty years in the local church. Would that I had been able to give this book to my parishioners in their time of need! Every pastor and church leader should have a supply of these books to give to anyone touched by cancer in their congregation. It may be the most impactful, effective, practical and spiritual tool any Christian leader can give to cancer patients and their family for pastoral care. Dr. Lane masterfully weaves godly wisdom and medical insights into a healing balm like that of Gilead!"

**-Dr. Larry Keefauver**

Bestselling Author and International Teacher

"We've all been touched by cancer: a family member, a close friend, perhaps even yourself. Rob Lane has served and cared for cancer patients and their families for decades, and over the years he has seen firsthand those he calls *Windrunners*, heroic souls who were able to, as Rob puts it, "stand up to the Dragon." In this direct and tender follow-up to his *Cancer's Bell Lap and The Dragon Behind The Door*, Dr. Lane shares their hope and their stories. This is not just a book for those affected by cancer, but is rather a companion of hope for anyone facing pain and suffering. But especially for those running that final *Bell Lap*, *Windrunners* will help you to discover that you are not alone, and that you've never been alone."

**-Chap Clark, Ph.D.**

Professor of Youth, Family and Culture, Fuller Theological Seminary, Author, *Hurt 2.0: Inside the World of Today's Teenagers*

"This book has provided this "Windrunner" a new perspective & study guide for developing a revised Home Stretch planning document for us and our four precious daughters. We are both in our 80's and are now armed and dedicated to fighting the Dragon as well as the bladder cancer as we approach the Home Stretch! We are eager to cram for Finals with the book's guidance to help us "Finish Well".

-**Barbie & Ken Hollingsworth**

# CANCER'S
# WINDRUNNERS

# CANCER'S
# WINDRUNNERS

*Spirit Powered*
*Hope Energized*
*The Dragon Vanquished*

## ROBERT F LANE, M.D.

XULON PRESS

Xulon Press
2301 Lucien Way #415
Maitland, FL 32751
407.339.4217
www.xulonpress.com

© 2017 by Dr. Robert F. Lane

Printed in the United States of America.

ISBN: 9781498493901

# DEDICATION

To all the Windrunners and most especially Wendell Price and Connie Jacobsen.

# ACKNOWLEDGEMENTS

The writing of this book has been my life for the past seven years and it is sometimes hard to trace back every idea and story to its original source. I attempt to do that in the notes at the end. The life stories you will encounter here are all true and most come from real patients and friends with their permission. Fictional names have been substituted for a few I could not reach or where the story is a conglomerate of several lives.

This book was made possible only through the guidance and encouragement of many friends and much prayer. I first want to thank my special friend and cancer survivor, Sue Wright, who devoted hours to teaching me from her own experience and to proofreading the manuscript through grace loving eyes, and to Mark Knowlden, Suzanne Kirsch, and Rick Enloe who labored through the roughest first draft and whose enthusiasm rescued it from the dustbin. With their guidance, we separated the practical and secular messages of the first book, *CANCER'S WINDRUNNERS*, from the spiritual and provocative messages of this book.

I owe so much gratitude to my mentors, Gino Grunberg, Rick Enloe, Chap Clark, and Larry Keefauver who helped me digest and integrate the great lessons from the Windrunners into a cohesive book.

I foremost want to thank my wife and sweetheart, Suzanne, without whose words of challenge and counsel and ever present encouragement this book would never have materialized.

Finally, I want to thank Larry Kefauver for his skillful and insightful copyediting to turn CANCER'S WINDRUNNERS into a more impactful book than I had written.

# TABLE OF CONTENTS

# PREFACE

# CANCER'S WINDRUNNERS

Cancer can be **defeated every time**, so **why** is it so terrifying for everyone?

It is because it attacks **the life you live**
    not just the body you live in.
It is because it attacks the life you live
    **more than** the body you live in.
It is because it affects most of the life you live **most of the time**
    while it attacks some of the body some of the time.

**It's not just about biology, it's about spirituality.**
**It's not about what is out of your control,**
**It's about what is in the center of your control!**

**Let the Windrunners show you how.**

I was jogging along Hood Canal on a hot August afternoon with a salt breeze in my face and the familiar scent of crushed madrone leaves underfoot. However, I was not feeling the familiar exhilaration of running: time alone, no phone, no schedule, no pain, just freedom, beauty, and a chance just to think. I had spent years focused on becoming a physician and NOW Three years out of training I was doing research, practicing hometown oncology, earning a living, but I was also totally bedraggled and beat up. Not burned out from working hours too long and too intense, but burned up because too many people were dying on my shift. No more than other oncologists, but still just too many. Cancer was winning JUST too often.

These were not just my patients; these were my friends. I knew their families and their dreams, and they knew mine. Together we had beaten back their disease, often several times; we had both celebrated and cried. No matter how many triumphs, there were just too many tears and too many deaths.

In training I had rotated from service to service, seldom seeing the same patient for more than a few months. Real medical practice was different because I was with the same patients for the long haul. There were lots of cures and remissions, but too often, the long haul became the final haul. That hurt... too much and felt like failure... too often.

For the first time while running along by the water, indecision struck. Maybe this is not what I am cut out for? Maybe I should do something different? What a miserable thought!

Being a man of some spiritual knowledge and a sometimes faith, I started to pray; something I had little experience with except in the foxholes of my life. I poured out my confusion and despondency to my sometimes God. Without remembering just what I said, I do recall with crystal clarity what He said, especially because I don't think I had ever heard Him say anything before.

**"I have got you exactly where I want you!"**

Startled and confused thoughts tumbled out. "Whoa! Where did that come from? Could that be God? What a presumptuous idea! Does God really speak out loud? And to guys like me?"

I concluded it just might be. A look around quickly revealed I was all alone and it sure wasn't me. At first I thought "that's cool," but then other thoughts flooded in. "What a bad idea. I don't like it and what does it mean?"

That is when I heard, **"It's not if they die; it is what happens before they die that matters!"**

**So I told him. It seemed to mean that everyone is going to die sooner or later and the timing was up to Him.** Yet, there also appeared to be something terribly important was supposed to happen first which was up to us. Apparently, my role could and should be more than I imagined, more than I had been taught. They were coming to me for treatment. Yet, at a more visceral level, they were coming for hope, and there was so much more to hope than just the medicine I was offering. I wasn't sure what it was and spent a few years sorting it out, but in that moment my focus shifted and expanded. I felt a sense of commission. Despondency seemed to disappear, and in its place came a new sense of purpose and possibility.

Thirty years later, and six months before my scheduled retirement, someone I had been getting to know awakened me at 3:00 A.M. with a compulsion, **"It is time to write what I have been teaching you."** Again, I thought it must be God because such an audacious idea was the furthest thing from my mind.

It happened twice before I finally got up and started to write. I knew it wasn't my voice or my idea because I had done everything in my science-focused education to avoid writing. This book is a testimony to the One who could distract me from all my beloved outdoor pursuits and plant me in front of a keyboard to write it.

The years and my patients have been hands-on teachers and their lessons have been profound. There was a group of patients beset by a tragic diagnosis whose lives refused to become tragic.

It was not because of what I did or what they did. Yet, invariably, they were victorious. I was astonished. Sometimes, they me told what they learned on their journeys; other times I learned from just watching them. Still other times, I learned in the dark and scary hours of my own journey.

## WINDRUNNERS

Something unique was going on with those patients. They were doing better than the rest and the Dragon was nowhere to be seen. You met the Dragon in the last book, *Cancer's Bell Lap and The Dragon Behind The Door,* and learned how it disabled so many people in both their lives and their fight against cancer.

It was a patient and a friend, Sue, who so eloquently described how the Dragon haunted her, and how she dealt with it. Since then, countless patients and even some non-patients have identified with Sue's experience with that metaphorical Dragon.

**"It would show up at the darnedest times, sometimes in the middle of the night and other times just as contentment or happiness was about to break out. There it was. Always a spoiler,"** she said.

They all described it as jeering voices in their heads of personal frailty or inadequacy, voices of the media fostering desire and discontent, and the voices of evil itself always whispering:

"You're going to miss out."

"Time is going to run out."

"What if?"

"Not enough."

"What if?"

And still more, "What if?"

No one could kill this Dragon, outrun it, hide from it, or cover it up with all kinds of beautiful stuff. Some were able to defeat it and run Bell Laps unhindered by it. What a mystery it all seemed. I had caught a glimpse of something true and have been in search of the fullness of that truth ever since. It wasn't their fitness, nor their ethnicity, nor the type or stage of their cancer. It was not their gender, age, education, or religion, but it was real, and it brought them peace and comfort amid turmoil and terror. Everyone at the cancer center could feel it and see it, but not pinpoint exactly what it was at first. Yet it set these patients apart. Despite the challenges of a Bell Lap, they ran like the wind inviting me to think of them as, "The Windrunners." (Yes, I have coined the word for this book and in honor of those remarkable people.)

None of us grow into spiritual maturity by choice. We're usually dragged there by suffering or enticed there by mystery. Most of us are spiritually lazy, willing to stay on the same path we're already on even if it is going nowhere. To find a new path takes motivation and daring. Windrunners had both, and it led to an unexpected adventure.

Often, it wasn't until the bell rang that anyone could sense the difference; most everyone smiles in happy-snappy land. The

Windrunners would generally separate from the pack right off the starting line, but not all of them. Some did not distinguish themselves until later. Something would change. They would move to the outside lane away from the Dragon, start pulling ahead of the pack in the backstretch, then fly round the far corner to join up with the rest of the Windrunners as they accelerated through the far corner and down the homestretch. Some are still running!

## THE EXPANDING SPECTER OF CANCER

There are more people being cured of cancer today than thirty years ago, but that is largely due to earlier diagnosis of localized disease for which surgery and other treatments are more likely curative. The cure rate for advanced stage disease hasn't changed much while our ability to keep patients in remission longer has improved. The number of people living under the apprehension of relapse and eventual death, both those hopefully cured and those unlikely ever cured, has grown enormously and without knowing it become Dragon fodder!

They all live on the outskirts of hope; ever feeling and fearing that there is a Dragon behind the door. For some, the Dragon is very big and others not so much. Some deal with it every day, others not so often. *They all know it is there.* It taints the lives of all but a few while manipulating decisions of most and stealing joy from all.

The Dragon is a problem bigger than most cancers and produces an *illness* of social, emotional, interpersonal, and spiritual chaos. It strikes at every cancer patient's heart, to wear away many a desire, erode many a dream, and even corrupt many a thought.

**Yet, some people can escape the hopelessness and deception. They not only defeat the Dragon, but smother it with irrelevancy by reframing the "what if?" question. They are the Windrunners.**

This book is about them, the exceptions to the norm, the ones who ran faster, further, with more grace, and often longer.

(Real life invariably brings some suffering which is curiously a prerequisite for engaging this book. If you are as yet unscathed, you may be too young to understand that. But cancer will change everything. If still unscathed, I would wait a few months to begin the book.)

*Who are they?*
*What makes their lives different?*
*What enables them to run their laps with such peace and purpose and even joy?*
*How is it they could finish so strong despite such a weakening and discouraging disease?*
*What does it take to be one of them?*

They are the people I have known, loved, and cared for who have run (or still are running) what might be their last lap and doing it really well! None seemed to know how long it would last. None had ever run it before or knew what to expect. None knew what pains and fears would lie ahead. None knew what resources they would have or what others would bring. None of them knew who would be with them and who wouldn't or how the disease would end. Yet they knew something and had something that enabled them to run like the wind anyway. Somehow, they seemed to know already that the planned obsolescence of our bodies, though it wears them out or breaks them down, is meant to transform us. They had already willingly begun that process.

*How do they do it?*
*Does it matter?*
*Can anyone do what they did?*

Their stories will tell you that it does matter immensely and that you can do it, too. It can be easy, but it is seldom obvious. It has to do with spirituality, but not in a way you might think, and not in a way that was obvious to me. I was missing something. I didn't understand what it was until a totally unrelated, serendipitous event occurred and God took advantage of it to instruct me. It involved something golden brown covered with fur, eight feet tall with a long nose, teddy-bear ears, and a large hump between its shoulder blades. I was about to face the bear—literally and figuratively.

# GUIDELINES FOR READING THIS BOOK

What I am sharing with you is garnered from the lives of patients, the crucible in which they were purified and clarified. It is said that an author must have two essential qualities for sharing—expertise and experience. Thanks to my professional training and the wonderful patients I have learned from, I hope that the truths we experienced together can be the fodder for such a process in you.

However, the banquet of ideas is so rich they cannot likely be digested all at once. Consuming too much, too fast can lead to much of it running right through you not leaving behind much of nutritional value. It needs to be consumed and contemplated in a piecemeal fashion. So while the chapters are topical and may be contemplated all at once for a reflective study group, I suggest you go through this book the following way

1.  You might want to skim over a whole chapter at first to get an overview of what's coming and then tackle one segment per day. If you need longer, take it. Don't rush. Journal and answer the questions.

2.  So, most chapters are divided into five segments or approximately five days. Read each segment and then stop. At the end of each segment is a journal page. On that page write down any notes or important truths you want to remember, memorize, and/or reflect/meditate on. If you need more space than this book has allotted,

then pick up a journal or empty notebook for gathering your thoughts, feelings, ideas, and truths.

3.  Yes, you are also writing a book for yourself and perhaps a family member or friend. I encourage you to not only read this book yourself but to do it with another person. The two of you may wish to discuss, share, speak truth in love to one another, and even pray for or with each other. I remember the proverbial truth, "There is a friend who sticks closer than a brother."[1] Another one reads, "A sweet friendship refreshes the soul."[2]

4.  Take time to go through each chapter. Let its truths go deep into your soul so that like fine food that must marinate, your memory is saturated by what is real, lasting, and even eternal.

Our memory is like a workbench for our projects, but there is limited space and the bench get smaller with stress and age. Each time another project or idea gets added others get bumped off unless there has been time to integrate the new idea with the database you have already stored in long-term memory files. The bumped off ideas are lost and forgotten. If you mull over the new information, it is more likely to be remembered and integrated. The ideas, facts, truths, and wisdom build on one another like

---

[1]  Proverbs 18:24b

[2]  Proverbs 27:9 MSG

individual Lego pieces creating a weapon that will vanquish the Dragon and beat the cancer.

# CHAPTER 1

# FACING THE BEAR

I was all alone 3000 miles north of my Seattle home when it came rambling rudely into my life. It walked right out of the fever dreams of my childhood and out of the Yukon tundra and taught me something that not only my cancer patients, but God had been trying to teach me for years – something the Windrunners already knew. Naked from a plunge in an arctic stream before making the dinner campfire, I came face to face with an animal drawn to the smell of food and looking for dinner.

*Any person has the capacity to learn profound things about oneself and God in a personal encounter with a horrible illness.* I had watched them for years on the cancer wards, but I was a slow learner until I met Ursus Actos Horribilis. My bare nakedness was no match for his bear grizzliness. While I quickly lost my appetite, that grizzly did not.

1

Only when I rounded a scrub fir carrying my shirt and shorts did I see my gun and clothes lying across my pack at the feet of a very large bear squinting at me through beady black eyes. Its head swayed from right to left as it studied me. ***I was without a weapon, a tree to climb, much of a plan or much of a faith. Odds of survival didn't look that good!***

I was caught completely by surprise, entirely vulnerable, defenseless, and alone; sort of the way cancer catches so many. I was cold with a clammy wetness and not just from the stream. My first inclination was to run, and so was my second.

***Why is it that prayer, conversation with God, is mostly limited in our lives to moments of desperation instead of regular times of intimacy?*** In the crisis of facing a bear, somewhere down my to-do list came the thought, *Pray!* Meanwhile, the bear just stood there getting bigger by the second, kind of like the dawning specter of a just-diagnosed cancer. Sound familiar?

***How very inconvenient it (any crisis) all was and how it spoiled all my plans.*** It interrupted what had been a marvelous day and promised to be a beautiful evening. Of course, I didn't think much about that; I was too busy just being scared. Much later, when the fear receded a little, I got really angry. That had more to do with getting my hands on a gun than being brave.

In the midst of that crisis, icy fear and intense anger took control. Thoughts of gratitude for still being alive were fleeting as fear and anger jockeyed for domination of my thoughts. How silly, ignoble, and arrogant of me to presume to be angry. The bear was only doing what bears do, following his nose towards food, and, in this case, me. ***Cancer just does what it does: grow continuously, invade, and then destroy other organs and lives.***

I am equally silly when I get upset with my body when it does what bodies do, i.e., break down. Dangerous and unpredictable *bears* will always appear in our lives, they just have different names. *The question isn't if crises (bears, dragons, diseases, etc.) will appear, but **when,** and **how** we will respond.*

**That bear taught me something that many learn from cancer, and it will stand me in good stead whichever terror I face next.**

Not many of us are as put together or secure as we think we are. Cancer can quickly reveal all the tiny cracks we are trying so hard to keep together. It can become an anvil on which so many lives are shattered, but that need not be the case. It does bring the key questions and obstacle of life into focus with great urgency for those paying attention.

In *The Bell Lap and The Dragon Behind the Door,* a cancer diagnosis became a metaphorical bell announcing possibly the last lap of a life. Not many recognize what that portends, neither the risks nor the opportunities, but those who do will address these key questions:

*Who am I?*
*Why am I here?*
*What has God got to do with it?*
*How do I run a better and often longer Bell Lap?*

# DAY 1

# A WINDRUNNER'S JOURNAL

*I invite you to reread every sentence above which is **bold** and in **italics**. Write it down, in your own words if you wish, to remember it, reflect on it, discuss it, or even memorize it.*

_____

_____

_____

_____

_____

_____

_____

_____

_____

_____

_____

## A Disease and an Illness

To begin to answer these questions, we need to understand cancer is both a disease and an illness. One affects your organs and the other your life. At first, you cannot detect either one until something vital stops working properly—either you hurt or your life hurts. ***The disease comes from injured genes, toxins or a virus, while the illness comes from something I call the Dragon. The doctors battle the disease, but it is up to you to deal with the illness and the Dragon.***

God has given us life and the right to dispose of it as we choose. Cancer does not lessen the number of choices, but it increases the urgency to get the decisions right. ***It will be your character choices about who you are and why you are here that will determine your destiny and your legacy as well as how happy you are along the way.*** No cancer can steal your character from you and no friend or doctor can give it to you. You don't need to be talented or wealthy, smart or strong, but you do need a good model and mentor. Who will be yours be?

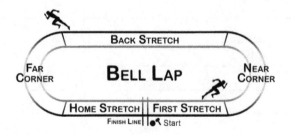

Both the disease and the illness, play out phase by phase over months and years. How does one grapple with two such foreign problems? The framework of running a race on an oval track and its Bell Lap helps us think sequentially about the phases of cancer and the strategies for living them. We dealt with a lot of the practical and medical aspects in the first book, but without including God in the equation. He doesn't want to foist Himself on anyone or be an obstacle for anyone in pursuit of practical knowledge, and I didn't want to do that for Him.

The cancer bell sounds to announce the beginning of what might be someone's final lap. Breathing hard down the first stretch, the cancer-scared runner reaches the near corner, endures treatment, and then rounds strongly into the remission backstretch. Relapse leads doggedly into the far corner which breaks breathlessly onto the home stretch ending graciously at the finish line.

The Dragon always appears on this lap and spews the very same life-altering, death-fearing illness into everyone's life sooner or later; if it is not already there. ***Cancer unmasks that Dragon by bringing it out in the open where we can see and experience the insidious drama of its actions.*** Everyone watching can recognize those who battle it victoriously and those who don't.

# THE BELL LAP AND THE DRAGON BEHIND THE DOOR

My first book addressed the planning and preparation necessary in the first stretch after hearing the Bell. Then it introduces the Dragon in the near corner with its many voices as well as the various tools and tricks it employs to trip us up as we are trying to collect ourselves for the treatment and a different life ahead.

*Those surviving that corner enter a backstretch of opportunity for spiritual reflection, discovery, and growth with an opportunity to optimize relationships and prepare to pass the batons of their life to the next generation.* The far corner is a time for tough and critical decision making. While the homestretch is for celebration and anticipation for Windrunners, it brings fear and dread for everyone else.

## WHERE DOES GOD FIT IN?

When the bell tolls, almost everyone at least fleetingly wonders, "What has God got to do with it?" Some set off on a spiritual journey which can make their Bell Lap as intensely a spiritual time as it is an intensely biologic, social, and economic time. Even those for whom everything spiritual smacks of hogwash start to wonder, "Does God have a role here? And, if so, how and what? Does it really make a difference?" Whether you are atheist, agnostic, Buddhist, Moslem, Hindu, or Christian, this time becomes one of dicey questioning, especially as you feel the heat of the Dragon's presence on the back of your neck and smell its breath.

*Cancer can destroy a body, but it often destroys a life first. A battle must be engaged on both the biologic and the spiritual fronts, recognizing that with every victory on one front frees up energy and resources to commit to the other.*

If my readers are anything like my patients, then I am speaking to a few who know God well, some who have just met Him, some who met Him long ago only to push Him onto a back shelf, some who were force-fed religion about Him only to walk away nauseated, and some who have never given anything spiritual much thought.

In the Cancer Center, I never knew to whom I was speaking, but I needed to speak to them all just as I want to with you right now. I have been in many of those same spiritual places myself and have wrestled with many of the same challenges. Please hang with me in those moments when I am writing to someone other than you. I believe there are some things, albeit different things, each of you will find meaningful, and beyond—essential and critical.

# Day 2

# A Windrunner's Journal

*I invite you to reread every sentence above which is **bold** and in **italics**. Write it down, in your own words if you wish, to remember it, reflect on it, discuss it, or even memorize it.*

_____

_____

_____

_____

_____

_____

_____

_____

_____

_____

_____

_____

_____

_____

_____

_____

# SCRIPT WRITING FOR ACT FOUR:
# THE BELL LAP

At first, I was like a fly on the wall watching my patients react suddenly to facing a bear called cancer up close and personal. Then, I became a like a narrator reading a story and watching a nightmare plot unraveling in their voices and on their faces. They wanted to wake up and find it was only a dream, but they didn't. So, I became an actor joining them on stage to act out a drama none of us had rehearsed.

*Now perhaps you or someone you love is on that stage, too, and you are discovering that the drama is about much more than just a disease. It is about what God wants and is waiting to do in your life which can now come into focus because of a disease.* It is what I think that voice whispering to me on my Hood Canal run was talking about. Cancer changes people.

"We would rather be ruined than changed. We would rather die in our dread than climb the cross of the present and let our illusions die."
-W.H. Auden

Most of us need to be cajoled, seduced or compelled to change. Renewal is invariably preceded by some sacrifice. It is almost the only pattern in legends and literature (real life and Scripture), but we don't want to see that because we don't want to change let alone give anything up. We're about getting more, not having or controlling less – until something falls apart like getting cancer and we have no choice. The upward journey requires some unavoidable stressor. "Falling down and moving up is, in fact, the most counterintuitive message of most world religions including and most especially Christianity."[3]

Not everyone is changed in any predictable way, yet surprisingly it is often for the better. *It was never the cancer biology that was beyond their control that made the difference. It was always something inside their control, in their hearts, minds, and decisions that did.* For some, it came easily and they fascinated me. Clearly they knew something and had something I didn't that I wanted, because deep down inside and seldom pondered, I feared I would be in their place one day.

I had my *bears*, but they were usually only in my dreams and almost always gone I when I woke up. However, I had seen so many awful diseases and injuries, so many lives altered in their prime, so many lives cut off just when the going was getting good, that I could not escape a gnawing feeling that tragedy would befall me someday and indeed it has.

---

[3]   Richard Rohr, *Falling Upward*, pg. xxii

So, I have watched, queried, and chronicled those friends and patients whose stories simply refuse to have tragic endings. Over the years, a picture has emerged and some truths have been revealed for me. I have put them to the test and they seem to be real. This book is about that picture and those truths that leap from the pages of my patients' lives. Let me show you the bread crumbs they left for us along the trail of their journeys through the dark forests of their cancers.

## SCIENCE OR FICTION

The scientific method taught in medical schools instructs us precisely what it takes to establish scientific fact. Research studies are performed under controlled conditions, evaluating a limited number of variables. The results are reported, reviewed, and published. However, one published paper of experimental findings does not a truth make. The methods of the experiment must also be published, the data evaluated, and then the same study must be reproduced by other reputable scientists in the same way, and must yield the same results. ***For me, it was as if my patients were doing a study with their lives and their souls. I was the scientist observing the consequences of their choices and was startled by the results.***

Now I think I understand their methods. I have passed them on to other patients, and I have tried them in my own life, and in both cases the original results have been reproduced. That is as close as I can get to the scientific method applied to the human condition, so I conclude the results are both valid and scientifically sound. When you finish reading, it will be for you to decide if it is just a bunch of hogwash or worth a try. Maybe your story is waiting to be part of a much bigger story.

# A WINDRUNNER'S JOURNAL

*I invite you to reread every sentence above which is **bold** and in **italics**. Write it down, in your own words if you wish, to remember it, reflect on it, discuss it, or even memorize it.*

_____

_____

_____

_____

_____

_____

_____

_____

_____

_____

_____

_____

_____

_____

_____

## You Can Do This

Some patients feel they have written every chapter of their lives carefully, tried hard, planned ahead, done everything right or at least done their best. Then along came cancer, presenting them with a chapter they have no idea how to write and their script comes to an end. They begin to flounder. For them, I hope this book will provide some clues and direction.

There are those who have had one hardship after another, after another, whose lives have been written by circumstances beyond their control. Once again an unfair, unjust author, this time named "Cancer," has taken up a pen in their lives. For them, I hope this book will show them a way to take the pen back and write their own story with both meaning and purpose, and an ending they are excited about.

This book is not meant to be a quick read. It is meant to offer both a map and a plan, but the map is more about topography than MapQuest directions, more about understanding the terrain and how to make strategic decisions than a roadmap of ready-made decisions. If you have cancer or some other life-threatening illness, you have suddenly discovered or it is slowly dawning on you, that you're quite lost in a world that is entirely foreign.

***Your survival depends upon navigating a landscape you have never seen before: the hospital corridors, operating rooms, MRI, and pet scanners.*** The fluids and the medicines are as foreign as the dark mountain woods. The people around you not only speak another language, but often with a cool dispassionate equanimity that is totally out of sync with what you feel.

Meanwhile, a voice inside your head is screaming, "This is **my** life we're talking about and I could die for Pete's sake." *You're lost in a biological nightmare with people who often seem to be emotionally disconnected. The fact that they have to disconnect just to survive what they do every day doesn't help you at all.*

When you're lost in the woods, you need to pay special attention to what's going on inside you as well as all around you. Is your urine getting darker yellow and less frequent; are you getting dehydrated? Are you still shivering, and are you thinking clearly or are you getting hypothermic? What does the sky tell you about the weather and the sun tell you about the points of the compass, and the flow the rivers tell you about the way out of the mountains? *You have to learn to read the terrain on the inside and the outside.*

I belabor this because those are the things most people don't think about until they're lost. They set off running in desperation to get safely home little realizing that speed has little to do with whether they survive let alone get out of the woods.

*Cancer is no different. In order to survive, you have to slow down and start thinking about the stuff you may have never needed or wanted to think about. You have to make observations about yourself, listen to your body, your soul, your past life, and consider all kinds of ideas, wrestle with them, and experiment with them.*

When you were a child, your world was small, and you didn't need to think about much at all. Mom and dad did that for you. As you grew, your world changed and you had to think about more things. Now your world has changed again big-time and more thought is in order. It's not as simple as, "Do what the doctor says, take this pill or that injection and everything will be fine." It won't. The bell has rung. You may be on your last lap, and there is a Dragon breathing down your back.

*Try to deny or dismiss the message of the bell and you will go down in a ball of flames like one of those World War II fighter planes spiraling to earth trailing smoke. Thinking takes time and must be intentional. So, take your time with this book, underline, scribble notes and questions in the margins and the journal pages. The battle must be won in your head first, so read until you're challenged then stop and wrestle with it for a while.*

You don't need to set aside any of your feelings. There will be anger, confusion, and depression because cancer is a profoundly unfair disease. I have felt them all, not only for my patients, but for my family as they have confronted leukemia, lymphoma, lung cancer, prostate cancer, and paralysis—some victoriously, some not.

**There is no easy way, but there is *an easier way, a way that is good*—even very good.**

***You have to believe in the possibility of what seems impossible in order to have any chance of reaching it.*** When an illness threatens your very life, it may seem impossible that living could still be full of purpose, meaning, joy, and even happiness, but it can. How could that be? We will explore that and learn from those who attest that it is true.

Throughout our lives, we encounter challenges that exhaust our physical and mental capacities. Common are the fleeting or not so fleeting thoughts, "I can't make it. I can't go on any further," that reverberate and can literally, on their own, defeat us. In reality they mean, "I've never gone this far before and I don't have experience to fall back on to encourage or guide me." I have seen this in patients' faces over and over again, and I have experienced it.

At the outset, I prepare them, and I get prepared. The Windrunners already are, but in more ways than we talked about in *The Bell Lap and The Dragon Behind The Door.* Before climbing mountains or sailing oceans, I used to read about people who have gotten into trouble and had to endure extraordinary hardships, been lost, injured, cold, hungry, and exhausted—at the end of themselves. I have wanted to know the limits of what others have endured and how they did it, so that if it happens to me I will have a reference point beyond my own suburban experience to nudge me onward with, "It has been done before, there must be a way. It can be done again; don't give up." *The preparation I am talking about now is spiritual and it takes every bit as much training— in your heart, in your mind, and in the field of everyday challenges of life—not just the book learning sort.*

I teach it to my kids, and I go with them to the edge of their endurance. With support, they learn not to be limited by their past experiences and that the battle for survival can be won. However, it has to be won in their heads first. It is the same with cancer. If you are dealing with a potentially fatal illness, it is unlikely that you have any past experience that will inform you of your own limitations, let alone how to go beyond them. *These stories can show you how people just like you have lived meaningful, exuberant, and purposeful lives despite the limitations of their strength, knowledge, and disease. I want to beckon you to follow them, get prepared, and start doing it now.*

This is a fragile and desperate time and nerves are raw. It can be hard to listen and digest all that you hear let alone put it all together. The temptation is to move too fast, listen too little, and think not enough. Preconceptions fueled by fear and anxiety misdirect the process.

# DAY 4

# A WINDRUNNER'S JOURNAL

*I invite you to reread every sentence above which is **bold** and in **italics**. Write it down, in your own words if you wish, to remember it, reflect on it, discuss it, or even memorize it.*

_____

_____

_____

_____

_____

_____

_____

_____

_____

_____

_____

_____

_____

## A FALSE PRECONCEPTION

The first preconception to dispel is that cancer grows fast and action must be taken quickly to attack it.

*With rare exception, cancer does not grow fast but it does grow relentlessly. Actions need not be taken quickly; rather they need to be taken thoughtfully and correctly. One set of decisions isn't right for every lifestyle. Therefore, take time to listen to your life, gather information, and rethink basic ideas. You have time to take a deep breath and make decisions carefully. It is your time to be thinking about some new things. Start now.*

> "Death is very likely the single best invention of
> Life. It is Life's change agent. It clears out the old
> to make way for the new." - Steve Jobs[1]

Richard Rohr elaborates on that idea noting that many of us remained stymied in the preoccupations of the first half of life: establishing a personal (superior) identity, creating various boundary markers for themselves, seeking security, and perhaps linking to what seems like significant people or projects. He asserts that while these are often good and necessary tasks, they "are no more than finding the starting gate" – the warm-up for the full journey. He notes that for many there comes a "crossover point" triggered by some "necessary suffering" which kindles a desire for something more, a larger reality, something akin to homesickness. If not ignored, a cancer diagnosis can create that crossover point. The 1st half involves the search for a life's script and multiple rough drafts. The 2nd half is writing and acting out the final draft, claiming it, owning it, and living into it. The perspective of years is often necessary to catapult one to change. This is not a luxury the cancer patient has. Recognize that a journey into the 2nd half of life awaits us all.[4]

I have wanted to write this book for a diverse group of people whose lives intersect with the ringing bell of the diagnosis. The most profound life-sustaining and life-expanding decision for many of them was to start, restart or accelerate a spiritual journey. While their motivations were similar and their destinations the same, the paths they took were markedly different. I recognize that you, like them, may be anywhere or nowhere along such a journey, so I have written from several different perspectives.

I will let the Windrunners' experiences speak for themselves. Where Christianity enters their stories, I have taken the input of patients, pastors, and theologians in an attempted to represent who Jesus is, how to know Him, and what difference it made. I try to do it through the lens of the faith experiences of my patients as well as my own, our stumbling blocks, and our "AH HA" moments, without presuming to be a seminarian or theologian. Rather than focusing on the nuances of doctrine that separates denominations, I've focused on the discoveries and practices that made a difference for those running a Bell Lap.

---

[4]  Richard Rohr, *Falling Upward*

To a layman such as me, any effort to describe God seems akin to that of blind men grabbing onto a different part of an elephant and trying to describe it. The descriptions have similarities but also differences, yet all are accurate in some way. One person has a hold of a leg, another has the tail, and another the trunk. When it comes to describing God in the cancer ward, I think I have got hold of at least an ear. I hope my words will give you enough accurate information to encourage you to grab on to the elephant yourself and discover more. Until then, I am a sojourner among others touched by cancer—more than most but not as deeply as some and now just seeking to compare notes.

# Time to Write the Rest of Your Life's Script

I am presuming you have read the first book and are equipped with a lot of practical ideas. If you have not read it, pause a moment. Get it. Read it. Also, continue reading this one as well. *With the first stretch and the near corner behind you, it is time for you to design the most important part of your Bell Lap and write your own script for the backstretch and far corner.*

**Better yet, let God write it.**

**If you do,** *you can be sure there'll be enough time to complete it.*

To do that, you have to journey intimately with Him for a while so start soon. I hope these chapters will help.

# DAY 5

# A WINDRUNNER'S JOURNAL

*I invite you to reread every sentence above which is **bold** and in **italics**. Write it down, in your own words if you wish, to remember it, reflect on it, discuss it, or even memorize it.*

_____

_____

_____

_____

_____

_____

_____

_____

_____

_____

_____

_____

_____

_____

# CHAPTER 2

# PEACE: THE ESSENCE OF A WINDRUNNER

*"There is the life we learn with and the life we live after that."*
– Glenn Close[1]

*"Disaster need not define your life, if you let it change you.*
*"* – Kyle Idleman[2]

I am often astonished by all the "what, why and how" questions of my children and often struggle to find the right words to respond. So, I resort to examples and stories that will convey meaningful answers they can comprehend. I learned that from the way God speaks to us in the Scriptures. When God reveals spiritual truths to us, he is limited to our language, as we are with our kids, and he too resorts to to metaphors and symbols. And yet we barely grasp what he is saying as "through a glass darkly" (1 Corinthians 13:12).

His parables intrigue our intellect, his ethereal music touches us deep within, the wonder of his beauty in the natural world fills us with awe, but none gives us the whole picture, the whole truth. But when we see the divine light shining through the life of a fellow human being in the midst of the ultimate peril, we know the whole truth must be out there and can be found and comprehended. That light draws us. It has drawn me as I have witnessed it in the lives of the Windrunners.

## CHANGE

*While immersed in the trial of our life, we are seldom able or even willing to see it as a time of learning or an opportunity for change*. Yet, cancer inspired one of my patients to go on a spiritual journey he never expected, and it changed his life. One day, he expressed the complicated feelings that remission created.

> *"It feels like re-entry into life, as if I have just returned from orbit where I could only dream about life and observe it from afar. With recovery, life feels different and curiously, I know I don't want my recovery to go too far. **I don't want to go back to the life I had before. I don't want to forget what I've learned. Knowing remission can end actually helps me hang on to what cancer has taught me.**"*

*"Days used to be filled with dreams, both good and bad, vacillating between the wonder of survival and the risk of recurrence. When risk commanded my attention, it did it so fully that the rest of life simply evaporated. Now, risk and wonder exist side-by-side. I don't like risk, but it has lost its power to terrify and control me because I know my God has wonderful plans for me on both sides of risk – plans I never knew before were possible. Even though I don't know what they are exactly, I am excited.*
***God's 'possible' has replaced my scary unknown - even my need to know.*** *I've seen His previews and I've heard His theme music. Whenever tomorrow awakens me in Heaven, it will be like walking into a dark theater filled with anticipation and having an amazing movie explode on the screen – only I will be in it!"*

He had joined the ranks of Windrunners running free, and it was all because of cancer. It is easy for a sceptic to disbelieve doctrine, but not to refute a changed life like his. I have never seen anyone rush to atheism in search of comfort and hope or to assuage their pain or fear of cancer. Whereas, many turn to God, fall to their knees, and start an ardent conversation with Jesus. Sadly, for many the conversation stops as soon as they are able to manage the pain just a little.

Not so with the Windrunners. There were many of them. Some blasted off the starting line when they first heard the Bell, some were already running hard when they got the diagnosis, while others had to collect themselves and look down the track before setting out. Some of the strongest runners stumbled, scraped their knees, and couldn't find their stride until they hit the backstretch. Others confessed that before they had been just plain stiff-necked about anything to do with God, but living so long under the shadow of death had transformed them. Then, there were some so overwhelmed by their cancer and its treatment that they couldn't think about anything else initially. They just hunkered down and endured the fear and the treatment, but it wasn't pretty. *Only when remission came, could they say, "Okay, Doc, what's that you said about a spiritual journey? I'm ready for it now." They had felt somehow exiled by distractions or injured lives, but now felt drawn toward a pilgrimage in search of a spiritual homeland.*

# DAY 1

# A WINDRUNNER'S JOURNAL

*I invite you to reread every sentence above which is **bold** and in **italics.** Write it down, in your own words if you wish, to remember it, reflect on it, discuss it, or even memorize it.*

_____

_____

_____

_____

_____

_____

_____

_____

_____

_____

_____

_____

_____

_____

## CROSSING THE THRESHOLD TO PEACE

*The first thing I noticed about the Windrunners was an ineffable peace in spite of all the fearful uncertainties that cancer delivered to their doorstep.* I could see it in their eyes, hear it in their voices, and see it in their lives. It seemed to be a place where they lived. It amazed me and I wanted it.

It had something to do with God, but it wasn't clear how they got there. It wasn't about just going to church, tithing, reading the Bible or getting dipped or dunked. It was something more. It seemed to be a profound knowing:

- *They knew God's promises for them and their families in this life and the next.*
- *They had given God a chance to prove His promises are real, that He is promise keeper, and trustworthy, and they were capable of trusting Him.*
- *They knew the principal obstacle on the track, the Dragon, and how to deal with it. Ultimately, they were able to live outside the bounds of time, beyond the jurisdiction, and reach of that Dragon.*

None were reaching for a target threshold when they crossed over, but the peace that arrived let them know they were beyond it. It was not something they sought or earned, but mysteriously arrived at while on a journey with Jesus. It was something different than book or head knowledge, but back then I didn't understand in what way, so I went in search of answers.

*Nary a Windrunner became one without first contending with a traumatic event somewhere in life which focused their attention on big questions. For some it was the cancer, while for others it had been earlier circumstances. Windrunners seldom came polished and shiny from happy-snappy land. More often they were bruised and battered from events that had shaken their worlds and tried their souls before they made the decisions that changed their lives.*

# DAY 2

# A WINDRUNNER'S JOURNAL

*I invite you to reread every sentence above which is **bold** and in **italics**. Write it down, in your own words if you wish, to remember it, reflect on it, discuss it, or even memorize it.*

_____

_____

_____

_____

_____

_____

_____

_____

_____

_____

_____

_____

_____

## NEW PATIENT CONVERSATIONS

When I first started talking to terrified patients about a place called peace, it didn't mean much to them. I had seen it in other patients' eyes, but they hadn't. Describing the Windrunners, who seemed to live in peace and how it enabled lives with purpose and even joy despite a guillotine diagnosis of cancer hanging over their heads, didn't get much traction. Many new patients already had a purpose which was to stay alive and they could get by without peace for a while to do it.

"Besides," one patient responded, "what is so special about peace? I'm not sure I have ever been at peace. There has always been something to worry about, but I have gotten by."

Over time their outlook often changed. After enduring a complete absence of serenity as their lives exploded with uncertainties, they often discovered a deep longing for something (call it peace) after all. By then, they had realized that their usual means of obtaining serenity weren't working; not even making new dreams, buying new stuff or taking new pills.

They started asking themselves, "What is it that I am lacking that causes me to be so unsettled? Why am I always reaching and searching?" Only then would they become interested in exploring, "Who is this God guy anyway? What's with this peace that passes all understanding?"

Some set out on a spiritual journey. Granting that death is an inevitable and natural part of life, one concluded that if an Almighty God created it, there must be a purpose behind it. Therefore, an implicit challenge for each of us is to figure out what it is. Some on that journey have since gone on to become a spiritual leader for their family and to inspire others even without a cancer journey.

*"If I hadn't been forced to stare death in the face, I would never have met Jesus and I would never have come to enjoy some of the simple pleasures in this life I have been missing. I have never been so content, so freed up from worry or so energized," said a guy who had been burned by religion and chased out of the church by dogma, parental expectations, and hypocrisy years before.*

There were some successful people who had been good at achieving goals on their own and felt the God-stuff was for lesser human beings. They just blew me off, and I left it at that. Curiously when disease progressed, some of them changed their minds and threw themselves wholeheartedly into exploring what faith and a relationship with Jesus was all about. However, with a late start their Bell Laps were short, less rewarding, and peace was only a puddle they splashed through rather than an ocean they swam in every day.

*It seemed that the Windrunner's peace was directly proportional to time spent with Jesus.* While a relationship with Him was purportedly not nearly as complex as a relationship with a spouse or teenager, it seemed to take time, commitment, and practice. The short lappers (those already looking death in the face) often just didn't have enough to figure Him out. Often perplexed, many still found their journey worthwhile as they discovered a new destiny in Heaven which delivered a calm to their final days.

Whichever way it happened, those who caught the wind of the Spirit finished stronger or are still running better. Surprisingly, there were not nearly as many as one might expect considering the thousands of patients I saw over the last thirty plus years even though the majority called themselves Christians.

***This goes directly to a central question of this book, and one I am frequently asked, "Don't all Christians deal with their cancer and the threat of death better?"***

It is always a hopeful question asked with a touch of anxiety, either by a humble Christian who isn't sure they are good enough or by a conceited one who takes their "Christianity" and salvation for granted saying, "Sure I believe in God, I'm a Christian, isn't most everyone?" Both are about to be surprised.

The truthful answer is, "No, Christians as a group don't deal with cancer or the threat of death better than non-Christians!" An incredulous, "Really? How can that be?" usually follows.

I spent a few years asking myself that question. Clearly, every Windrunner I met was a Christian and yet there were others who called themselves Christians, even some clergy, who were stumbling all over the track, clearly not running well at all, fraught with fear, and clearly not experiencing "the peace that passes all understanding."

I couldn't just tell patients, "Here are the four spiritual laws, now go to church, confess, submit, catch the wind, run, and you will be fine. See you in Heaven." Most of my patients who did that were not fine and I don't know about Heaven yet. I do know they could jog, but never run and often complained they could feel the heat of the Dragon, fear and worry, coming up behind them.

*So what was different about Windrunner Christians? Their journey did begin with meeting God, so let's start there and then ferret out just what it is that enables some who meet Him to live such amazing lives, even in the valley of the shadow of death.*

# DAY 3

# A WINDRUNNER'S JOURNAL

*I invite you to reread every sentence above which is **bold** and in **italics**. Write it down, in your own words if you wish, to remember it, reflect on it, discuss it, or even memorize it.*

_____

_____

_____

_____

_____

_____

_____

_____

_____

_____

_____

_____

_____

_____

_____

## WHAT'S WITH MEETING GOD?

When patients were coming out of the near corner, induction chemotherapy behind them, in remission or not, I started recommending that it might be a good time to consider a spiritual journey. I was met with a variety of responses from, "I'm already on one" to "been there, done that, what a bunch of BS" to "I went to church as a kid, not sure why I stopped, going back now seems like a good idea" or "What's that? What's being a Christian like?" That last one caught me off guard. My confidence as a physician didn't extend to leading someone spiritually as I was just getting to know God myself. I kind of knew where they needed to go, but not how to get there.

I suspected it started with the alleged son of God. One does not even need to believe in his divinity to realize that Jesus is seeing at a much higher level than most of us and is the spiritual authority of the Western world, whether we follow him or not. Not knowing much else, I took a quick sidestep and told them here's what others told me."

**Elizabeth:** *"For me, believing was a choice, not just a one choice, onetime deal. First, I chose to become open to the possibility of believing.* An 'Okay God, God, I'm open, show me' sort of thing. I started reading the Bible and listening to others' experiences with God, then it seemed events unfolded, ideas seemed to crystallize in my head, then they sort of incubated for a while like the ingredients in bread dough, taking on new shapes, and getting bigger. My priorities and even my actions started changing and I liked it. Then one day I realized I was starting to believe. I think when I opened the door a crack to the possibility of God, His Spirit came in like yeast and pulled the ingredients together and then I experienced belief growing. But I had to choose over and over to invite Him into my world and, when I did, I discovered this God thing was a whole lot bigger than I thought at first."

**Ben** was the agnostic son of a Presbyterian preacher. He knew every academic argument for faith and had an academic rebuttal for each. He described himself as a "Nowhere Man!" When he got cancer he told me he felt, "Lost, adrift, and afraid." For the first time since childhood he prayed. He said it was like a J-PEG download of the old sterile God-stuff from his adolescent brain to his adult heart. *The information hadn't changed, but everything else had. "I never believed in the cosmic invisible God in the sky until He met me in the depths of my pain and I could feel His presence." Against the backdrop of the life he had lived, all of a sudden it made sense, it felt different, and it made a difference. "My life has changed in ways I would never have imagined, ways that I just plain rejected before. I am amazed!"*

**Christopher** told me that God invites us into a theater of great expectations where commitment is the only price of admission. Once paid, each attendee gets a new pair of glasses, sort of like those yesteryear 3-D ones. Nothing changes on the screen of life, but our perceptions and understanding does. We start to see another dimension of reality through God's eyes. When we do, our behavior changes, not as a function of arduous discipline, but because seeing things differently leads to different desires and decisions. We hope more, but in a different direction and expect it to happen.

**Charlie** said he attended church occasionally because it made his wife happy, but he was pretty turned off by some hypocrites there who called themselves Christians. Then he realized that not everyone given a fishing rod catches fish and everyone who hears the music can dance, but that doesn't change the truth about the existence of fish in the stream or the rhythm in the music. When he concluded that he had made a mistake by confusing the wannabe Christians with Jesus Himself, *Charlie felt free to get to know the real Jesus. "I think I had a faulty mental model of who Jesus is and as a result I couldn't see Him even when He was right in front of me. Talking to people who had never met Him, but thought they had, didn't help. They just sent me on the wrong course."*

**Margie** described how through the years she had become completely "churchified" then bagged it all. When I asked her what she meant by that, she explained that her faith had been wrought with obligations, should-haves, shouldn't-haves, better-nots, shame-on-you-ifs, but never about getting to know Jesus. She told me she had confused her church with God Himself and had been marching to the music instead of dancing with God, and then she rejected both. It was not until she realized that the church, though well intentioned, remains a human creation, and as such, sometimes falls short of God's intention that she was able to reconsider either one.

She had found herself another church which nourished and inspired her and actually introduced her to Jesus. When that happened, she said it felt like a load was taken off of her back and replaced by an upwelling of passion in her heart. "Want-tos" replaced the "better-nots." Passion about the things that matter to God replaced the dread of breaking God's alleged rules.

***It didn't happen all at once. She needed to stand in the doorway of every room of her life, fling open each door, and invite Jesus in. Then she quoted Ezekiel 36:26–28, "I will give you a new heart and put a new spirit in you; I will remove from you your heart of stone and give you a heart of flesh. I will put my spirit in you and move you to follow my decrees."***

**Carol** thought she had "PTFD" (Post Traumatic Faith Disorder). When she looked back at the last few miserable months of her life, she realized that her suffering was tempting her to doubt her faith. It didn't make sense. All along, she had had faith in the goodness of God and then she came face-to-face with cancer. Whenever she had observed others suffer, she had assumed they didn't really know Jesus the way she did. She had learned from the Bible to expect suffering and she had read Jesus' words, "Blessed are they that mourn," but somehow she had expected that if she stuck close to God she would dodge the strife. When she started to experience real suffering and really suffered, she began to wonder if her faith was real, if God was real, thinking maybe it was all imagined, maybe just wishful thinking.

She realized how easy it had been to sign up for salvation and to experience the joy of worship, but now she wondered whether it was all a charade. It had come so easily at first, but once cancer came, the world turned dark and doubt was everywhere. Later, God had come to her in the darkness and helped her pick up the pieces of her faith that, "had collapsed all over the floor like a house of cards blown down."

She couldn't begin to tell all that she had learned, but she did say that without her suffering her eyes and heart would not have been opened to where God really wanted to lead her. It was as if the wounds of her cancer were the windows that let God's light shine in deeper that it had ever penetrated before. ***Now she knew beyond a shadow of a doubt in her heart, God loved her.*** She knew He was not the cosmic sadist she had called Him. If there had been any other way than suffering to teach her, He would have provided it and He wouldn't have had to tell her to expect it.

*Now He was calling her out of her suffering to a new purpose. It was a purpose outside of herself that in spite of her illness, lifted her life out of the doldrums of focusing on her own limitations. She found in scripture evidence that those who suffer greatly but nobly will enjoy a greater capacity to serve God in heaven (see Philippians 2:8, Matthew 20:20–23, Romans 8:18, 1 Peter 4:13). That encouragement, she shared, "Called my thoughts out of the present and into the future, away from*

***the physical into the spiritual and toward a purpose beyond the temporal into the eternal."***

**Steve** was in ministry with high school and college students before beating his metastatic testicular cancer with aggressive chemotherapy. I watched him engage them saying, "Becoming a Christian was like joining a basketball team and listening to the radio." Quirky but it caught their attention and mine.

Then Steve asked them how that could be. Most were quiet until one kid piped up, "Well, you can't very well play basketball by yourself." Steve agreed Christians do better in groups where they can support, encourage, and learn from one another. The exchange continued. They ferreted out that in both basketball and Christianity you can sign up and then learn the game from others or an instruction book. Then you can learn to talk the game or God pretty well. You can wear the jersey and feel pretty cool, but the real deal doesn't start until you get on the court and start practicing what the coach says. It's not easy and it doesn't come naturally for many, but the coach, just like Jesus, is right there to offer advice on every move and shot, confusion or aggravation.

"So what is not easy about Christianity?" he asked. They responded, "It's hard to listen to God especially in the moment, when life is full-on happening." That brings us to the point about listening to the radio," Steve prodded. No one got it, so he explained that we are always listening to thoughts in our head. We wake up in the morning and on goes our thought radio which is almost always tuned to KMF (Kinda Me First). It is tuned to my agenda: what is easiest and best for me. But no one ever hears God's voice on that channel. He will speak into the thoughts in your head, but only if you switch channels to KGW (Knowing God's Will) and listen very carefully. The volume is often low, so low that it's easily drowned out by the static in the rest of our lives."

*Steve continued, "You may have to slow down to listen, because you will never hear Jesus at high speed. He requires your full attention. He doesn't want to thwart your will; He just wants to guide it, but only if you are interested." It seems Steve was talking about connecting with the Holy Spirit. I thought Steve was pretty random, but clever. Maybe that's what it takes to connect with kids and keep their attention.*

# A WINDRUNNER'S JOURNAL

*I invite you to reread every sentence above which is **bold** and in **italics**. Write it down, in your own words if you wish, to remember it, reflect on it, discuss it, or even memorize it.*

_____

_____

_____

_____

_____

_____

_____

_____

_____

_____

_____

_____

_____

## WHAT SEPARATES WINDRUNNERS FROM THE REST?

**Peter:** "I've met God but I don't have the peace that you are describing. What is so different about these so called Windrunners and how did they do better?" queried a man with salt and pepper hair in a grey pin striped suit, polished cap-toed shoes, and a newly diagnosed kidney cancer.

It seemed that irrespective of where they were on the track, the Windrunners awakened to yet another sunrise and saw it as a gift and as evidence that Jesus still has plans for them on this side of eternity even in spite of cancer and maybe something for which the cancer would uniquely prepare them. They saw it this way because they really seem to **know Him,** not just know **about Him.** Even more than that, they really seemed to **trust Him.**

I would always hesitate to say that, because the usual patient response spoken with their eyes if not their words was, "Yes, sure Doc, but what about the cancer?" With that rejoinder, I would counter with, "It's all about the cancer, so hang with me. Let's take it one step at a time."

# Time to Write the Rest of Your Life's Script

In order to continue to write the next phase of your life's script, you have to want to study and learn from the Windrunners. The first thing I noticed about the Windrunners was an ineffable peace in spite of all the fearful uncertainties that cancer delivered to their doorstep. It wasn't about just going to church, tithing, reading the Bible or getting dipped or dunked.

It seemed to be a profound knowing:

- They knew God's promises for them and their families in this life and the next.
- They had given God a chance to prove His promises are real, that He is promise keeper, and trustworthy, and they were capable of trusting Him.
- They knew the principal obstacle on the track, the Dragon, and how to deal with it. Ultimately, they were able to live outside the bounds of time, beyond the jurisdiction, and reach of that Dragon.

*Which of the above do you know that you know?*
*Which ones have you yet to discover?*
*How did the Windrunners get to the place where they could trust God?*

*Did they have to become passive?*
*Did their lives have to become dull and boring without dreams*
*or passions?*
*Did they need to surrender being themselves?*

**Let's now find out what sets the Windrunners apart from
others and how they achieved this empowering trust in God.**

# A WINDRUNNER'S JOURNAL

*I invite you to reread every sentence above which is **bold** and in **italics**. Write it down, in your own words if you wish, to remember it, reflect on it, discuss it, or even memorize it.*

_____

_____

_____

_____

_____

_____

_____

_____

_____

_____

_____

_____

_____

_____

# CHAPTER 3

# THE TRUST THAT POWERS WINDRUNNERS

I didn't recognize them at first because I had no idea there was such a thing as a Windrunner, or for that matter a Bell Lap until I saw someone running for their life and doing it well. No one had told me about them in medical school, on the evening news or from the pulpit. Then I met one, and saw one, then another, and another.

Who were these people and what was so special about their stride? They had been there all along, but I had never recognized them until that life-shattering sound of the bell rang out in their lives, that life threatening diagnosis of a possibly race/life ending disease.

Many Windrunners took a stutter step, some even stumbled to the ground, but none stayed down or ran away, and none pretended they hadn't heard the bell. They knew they had to deal with the same stuff as everyone else who hears the bell. They still ran headlong into all the confusing times of testing and diagnosis in the first stretch and near corner, the hard times of trying to understand the medical environment and start treatment, the same devilish adversaries of fear and false hopes, and they all had to consider descending into denial or defeat or bargaining for grace. ***Somehow, the Windrunners recovered their stride or never lost it, but came powering out of the near corner pulling ahead of the pack.***

Some distinguished themselves early right out of the blocks, but all were catching the attention of every onlooker by the time they lengthened their stride and moved into the outside lane of the backstretch when the diagnosis and prognosis were complete, the treatment started, and a new life with a new disease was coming into focus.

I could see they were running strong and distancing themselves from the others, with less fear, less angst, more joy, and more purpose. Something special was going on, but what? Clearly they were better prepared, yet none had known the bell was about to ring. How could that be? There were dozens of them, but not hundreds amid the thousands I cared for.

*A consistent theme that united
Windrunners was this: they were all
running toward God rather than away
from death.*

I will tell you about Becky, Fred, Chuck, Connie, Gale, Lisa, Sally, Jim, Dave, Mary, Karina, Doris, and Al, but FOR NOW let me tell you about Wendell Price.

**Wendell** was the first of what I was later to recognize as Windrunners. He came in on a Friday afternoon with his wife, Muriel, complaining of feeling tired. He was fifty-seven years old, trim and athletic, but too pale for a guy with Polycythemia Vera, a disorder in which the bone marrow makes too many red blood cells usually producing a super healthy, ruddy complexion. It hadn't given him much trouble apart from the hassle of HAVING A PINT OF BLOOD REMOVED occasionally. Now it looked like he didn't have enough – how strange – not good. Yet, on that day, little bothered him except a little breathlessness on his usual three-mile run.

Physical and laboratory examinations were normal except he was a little pale and a little anemic. Blood under the microscope told a different story; myeloblastblasts were present. These cells are supposed to live only in the bone marrow and come out into the blood stream only under extraordinary biologic stress, which he clearly did not appear to be experiencing, or if a terrorist plot hatches inside the bone marrow.

That was exactly what was happening. One myeloblast cell had somehow been injured or mutated causing it to start reproducing itself in an entirely uncontrolled fashion, thereby disobeying every norm of respectable cell social behavior. Its progeny were taking over the bone marrow and displacing all the other normal marrow cells including the ones needed to carry oxygen, fight infection, and clot the blood. Then the criminal offspring myeloblasts overflowed into the blood to spread to other organs.

Wendell never saw it coming, but AML, Acute Myelogenous Leukemia, had just arrived, which in 1982 was a virtual death sentence.

Distraught for them, I began to describe the catastrophic news of his diagnosis. There were only three medical care options. If he took no treatment, he would probably only survive a few weeks. If he took some relatively non-toxic chemotherapy that could be given in the office, the growth of the leukemia might slow down enough that he might survive an average of three months. Alternatively, there was a third option: he could be admitted to the hospital immediately and started on the best, albeit very toxic, chemotherapy which offered an 80 percent chance of complete remission (average survival of two years) and a long shot chance of cure.

That treatment would initially involve four to six weeks of hospitalization with significant chemotherapy toxicity and about a 10 percent chance of dying soon in the process. If the treatment was successful at inducing remission, it would be followed by multiple similar hospitalizations for complex cycles of chemotherapy over the course of a year. I told him that despite the arduousness of such treatment, option three is exactly what everyone under the age of seventy had always chosen.

Wendell listened closely. For a moment it seemed that all the oxygen sucked out of the room; no one even breathed. Eyes search the corners of the ceiling. Time seemed suspended for a moment and then he looked me square in the eye and spoke, *"I know two things: my life's verse is Philippians 1:6, 'He who has started a good work in me will complete it by the day of Jesus Christ.' And the cool thing about that is God is not limited by any human timeframe. He just promises to do it. Period. But there is a caveat. For me to claim that promise I need to walk into my God-given calling – give Him a chance to lead, then follow or He will have no opportunity to finish what He has started."*

Then he told me that his calling was to be on the pulpit[1] of the church up the street every Sunday, "So Doc, give me the best stuff you got that will get me on that pulpit in two days and every Sunday thereafter for long as possible."

Flabbergasted, I figured he hadn't heard what I had just said; many people don't hear anything after I say the words "cancer "or "leukemia." So, I explained again how the arduous treatment was really the only one of significant possible benefit and it would entail his being in the hospital for several weeks and missing several Sundays, but it stood the best chance of getting him on the pulpit for more Sundays in the long run, i.e. give up six to twelve Sundays now and get ninety or more later.

*Then he pointed out,* **"God's promise in Philippians has nothing to do with time. It is outside time."**

That is exactly where it seemed to me Wendell was stepping and I was clueless - definitely outside my training and life experience.

*Wendell was certain that God would complete his life*
*in meaningful and wonderful ways*
*in whatever time there was left.*
***It was God's responsibility to figure out the timeframe.***

Wendell wasn't going to interfere with that or worry about it. Instead, he was going to get on with his calling. As I bargained with him, he looked me in the eye and countered with, **"I would rather trust God's promises than doctors' statistics."** I was pretty much jaw-dropped speechless at that point. There was no fear present, not a hint of that sulfurous dragon breath.

So, I gave him the mild chemotherapy in the office thinking it was little more than a placebo and pretty soon I started seeing what a Windrunner looks like. There was no wild spiritualizing, no touting God's grace, love, and power, and no boasting about his own faithfulness and commitment, no claiming what God owed him or how God was certain to rescue him. He simply went on with his family life, loving his wife and raising his daughters and son, and with his ministry, but with even more intentionality and purpose. *There was a peace about him I could little fathom or understand. It seemed like the cares of this world blew by him without ever breaking his stride, altering his focus or tarnishing the quiet smile on his face.*

# Day 1

# A Windrunner's Journal

*I invite you to reread every sentence above which is **bold** and in **italics**. Write it down, in your own words if you wish, to remember it, reflect on it, discuss it, or even memorize it.*

_____

_____

_____

_____

_____

_____

_____

_____

_____

_____

_____

_____

_____

_____

## INADEQUACY AND VULNERABILITY

All of life has a way of pointing out our inadequacies often getting help along the way from parents, spouses or employers. A cancer diagnosis adds one more voice of incrimination to that storehouse of brokenness, shame, and guilt that we try to keep hidden or disguised. Some facing cancer play a charade of continuing all of their usual activities for as long as possible, as if nothing has happened. Some are brash: "It's no big deal. I'm going to beat it" or "God will cure me." Others just hide. Not so for Wendell.

*If cancer makes one feel defective, the first impulse can be to seek refuge by disengaging from relationships, responsibilities, hobbies, and new endeavors, but that has a cost. There is loss of connectedness with those who can validate, love, and encourage; even loss of self-worth and identity. Not so with Wendell. He chose a path of even greater engagement, daring to share the challenges and dangers he faced right from the pulpit and with everyone he encountered.*

He was a leader and leaders are supposed to be strong, but he chose a different kind of leadership. No false bravado, no cover-up, no righteous posturing. Right when illness was producing inescapable weakness, instead of hiding, he became more vulnerable and authentic with everyone and they loved him. In the face of physical uncertainty, risk, and peril, his confidence in God's purpose and provision shown through. It inhabited his preaching and amplified his words. Lives around him changed. The strength and courage to acknowledge those painful, frightening feelings endeared him to people and increased his credibility, but where did they come from?

*He told me it was not about bravery; it was about <u>trust</u>. He confessed that the first time he trusted Jesus to direct his steps, inhabit his circumstances, and mold his heart, it took courage, but now that he had done it so many times, confidence had replaced the need for courage.*

*He had come to trust God's plan – a plan that was beyond time and beyond imagination, and that trust had become unshakeable. It showed! Peace dwelt in his life.*

We met each week. I was the doctor who relied on my hands, but he was the healer who touched my heart and opened my eyes. He tutored me with his life and when I asked questions, he used words. I probed. Where did the passion come from, that fire in the belly that energized this quiet but committed man? It was a mystery to me. He told me it had to do with the Paschal Mystery – the what?

As what I learned gained depth and breadth, I started seeing it in other patients who were running Bell Laps with the same amazing grace that I had seen in Wendell. It was as if something lifted them off the ground above the friction of everyday concerns and propelled them forward. *It was Wendell who told me it was the wind of the Spirit, and while I wasn't really sure what he meant, I could see it in action. Hence, the name Windrunners that I have been using ever since.*

# DAY 2

# A WINDRUNNER'S JOURNAL

*I invite you to reread every sentence above which is **bold** and in **italics.** Write it down, in your own words if you wish, to remember it, reflect on it, discuss it, or even memorize it.*

_____

_____

_____

_____

_____

_____

_____

_____

_____

_____

_____

_____

_____

## TRUST EXPERIMENTS

*May the God of hope fill you with all joy and peace as you **trust** in him, so that you may overflow with hope by the power of the Holy Spirit.* (Romans 15:13)

*"Trust building must first take place with the little things in the good times if you expect to have it for the big things in the bad times."* - Unknown

For Wendell, running like the wind was all about trusting Jesus. That is the foremost thing that sets the Windrunners apart, but there is more to it than it would seem at first. Believing Jesus is trustworthy is not enough; a desire to trust Him is not enough; even a decision to trust Him is not enough. They are all essential, but not enough. The kind of trust Wendell was talking about is possible for anyone, but it takes practice and it is incremental. It takes time to build and it requires accumulating personal evidence that can only happen through a series of trust experiments.

***To trust you have to know.*** Knowledge is either academic or experiential and that applies to God as well. Learning about Jesus from scripture or sermons is useful, but learning who He is by experiencing Him is critical.

*Learning about Jesus may inspire you to believe, but only experiencing Him can inspire you to trust.*

In the gospel of Mark, a father brings his epileptic, mute, deaf, and demon possessed son to Jesus imploring Him, "If you can do anything. Take pity on us and help us." The man obviously knew enough about Jesus to *believe* He was a healer, and had enough *hope that* Jesus would indeed heal his son, but something was missing. Jesus responds, "If you can? Everything is possible to the man who trusts." The father responds, "I do believe! Help my lack of trust" (Mark 9:23-24 NASB), "Help me with my unbelief" (NIV), "Help me with my doubts" (MSG).

The father had never had an opportunity to risk trusting Jesus or put his belief into action before. He had been only a passive observer of Jesus and the recipient of hearsay evidence about Jesus – just like the rest of us. We hear about Jesus. We read about Jesus. We may even see Jesus in the actions of others. That is only knowledge AND IT IS ALL PASSIVE. It cannot become truth until we appropriate it for ourselves and act on it by seeking Him and risk following His lead. Then knowledge can become experiential, foundational, and becomes truth. Then it becomes ours! Until then it is someone else's. When it becomes ours, trust begins and only then can it be built upon to become powerful in our lives.

It is easier to believe and to act in accord with someone you trust. It takes an encounter, an interaction, risk, trial, error, discovery through experiential knowledge, and being with them to build that trust.

*Take heed: it is only through practicing trust with God that builds an enormous trust and that is what eliminates anxiety. Trusting Jesus is the road to peace.*

It starts with belief in Him which leads to hope and emboldens risk. Together they empower the traveler toward trust. Trust is not a whistle-stop destination. It is a mountain to be climbed, one trust step after another until the panorama of peace explodes before you at the summit. From there you can see everything more clearly, both where you have been and where you are going. Then it all starts making sense.

You don't need to climb alone. Given the opportunity, the Holy Spirit finds its way into all your inner worlds of strife and blindness and beckons you to take sides with Jesus against your own areas of darkness and defeat. *In the words of C. Baxter Kruger and W.P. Young, take "incremental steps of trust and change."*[24]

*Stepping out in trust starts with asking Jesus for advice in decision-making, for His Spirit to influence your attitudes, His divine insight to aid understanding, His strength to power endurance, or His behind the scenes action to influence events around or inside you.*

*Trust steps start out just walking and with perseverance they become running.* Then like those diving ducks that run across the surface of the water before taking to the air, you, too, can experience lift off. With the mysterious power of God beneath your wings, you defy the gravity of grief and rise above the concerns of this world that want to drag you down. The concerns are still there, but they lose their grip on you.

If you haven't experienced trust, these words may sound pretty bizarre, but it is exactly where the Windrunners live. Worldly concerns still tug at them, but their tether has been broken, their control lost. It's sort of like Peter on the Sea of Galilee who was able to defy gravity and walk on the water as long as his eyes were fixed on Jesus and walking toward Him (see John 6:16, Mark 6:45, Matthew 14:22). He trusted Jesus who beckoned him out of the safety of the boat onto the waters he feared. Peter trusted someone he had not just met or heard about, but someone he had lived with, intimately conversed with, and come to trust.

Recall that Peter began to sink into the water when he took his eyes off Jesus and became distracted by the storm. ***Cancer and the aggravations of the world around you will try to distract your attention from Jesus and His calling. It is not easy to maintain your focus; it is a moment by moment, day by day thing which takes practice. Only staying connected to Jesus will keep building the trust and confidence that lets you walk over the waves and through the storms in peace. The Spirit wants to help you do it.***

# DAY 3

# A WINDRUNNER'S JOURNAL

*I invite you to reread every sentence above which is **bold** and in **italics**. Write it down, in your own words if you wish, to remember it, reflect on it, discuss it, or even memorize it.*

_____

_____

_____

_____

_____

_____

_____

_____

_____

_____

_____

_____

## BE A SCIENTIST

If you bother to read the instruction manual for your new cell phone, you will learn all the cool things it can and cannot do. You learn it doesn't work well as a hammer or as a can opener and don't get disappointed when you can't hang a picture or open a beer with it. If you just started pushing buttons, you will probably make some mistakes, but eventually will figure out how to make a call. However, you won't discover many of its cool apps described in the manual.

It's the same way with God. No reason not to jump right in with every prayer need, but don't be surprised if the answers are different than what you hope for. You can pray all you want for new Porsche in the driveway or diamond/sapphire earrings on the dresser, but a quick glance at God's Bible will save your breath. If you start reading it you will not only get a better idea of what His answers will be, but you'll also get an idea of His amazing apps.

There is very little we trust without testing it first or at least getting an endorsement from someone who has tested it. Even getting into a new car we checked the steering and brakes at low speed before putting the pedal to the metal. Getting on a horse, we put it through its paces to learn what to expect and to build our confidence before taking it into the mountains. God knows we are built this way. He expects no less. He does expect us to check Him out and doesn't expect us to get it all right at first nor ever require it. He already knows how much less than perfect we are and just hopes we will try.

*You first need to know who He is so you can know what to try and what to expect when you do.* We don't get on a horse and expected it to fly just because Pegasus did. We expect a horse to do what horses do. God will only do what God does and He works in mysterious ways; wise to learn about those before asking favors based on false expectations.

*Checking references is common practice before hiring someone and it should be done with Jesus before giving Him your life.* Start with Matthew, Mark, Luke, and John, the first four books of the Bible's New Testament. They will give you time tested, Holy Spirit inspired, first and second hand accounts of what Jesus actually said and did 2000 years ago. Then read accounts describing what Jesus is doing in the lives of people today. (I'll give you some.) Then talk to people in whose lives Jesus is at work right now. While we often know those around us who walk with God, we seldom know their stories and what God has done in their lives nor what they have ask of God and how He has responded. So ask them.

*Be selective who you question.* Choose someone who has been walking with God a while. Beware of those who have tried and failed. They clearly haven't figured out who Jesus is and lacking that, their expectations have probably been off base and disappointing. Disgruntled, they will be quick to tell you it can't be done and isn't worth the effort. They are often the ones who asked questions expecting God to be their Genie and were disappointed. God doesn't do the Genie thing. He does the God thing. It's best to understand what that is before you go asking Him for His help. Then be scientific about it.

For any experiment in a scientific laboratory or in the laboratory of your life, there must be an astute and patient observer who is looking for results – not only the ones he expects, but for any and every result. The scientist needs to be open to whatever the results may be and willing to reevaluate the original assumptions that the results failed to validate. He must then be willing to build on the results to create the next experiment.

*That is precisely what one needs to do with God. Every experiment is an investment in your relationship with Him and every trust experiment teaches you more about who He is. Each improves your ability to hear His voice and see His hand moving in circumstances all around you. However, trust experiments are about more than just discovering who God is, they are about discovering if you are who you think you are and profess to be!*

I am not talking about getting religion and moral perfection with an expectation that it will help you with your cancer. Marching to the drum of purity codes, avoiding the "thou shalt nots" or preaching from the corner or even the pulpit will not take you where you need to go–down to your knees with an open heart (2 Corinthians 12:10 "...when I am weak, I am strong").

# Day 4

# A Windrunner's Journal

*I invite you to reread every sentence above which is **bold** and in **italics.** Write it down, in your own words if you wish, to remember it, reflect on it, discuss it, or even memorize it.*

_____
_____
_____
_____
_____
_____
_____
_____
_____
_____
_____
_____
_____
_____

# EXPECTING GOD TO BE GOD LEAVES HIM ROOM TO SURPRISE YOU

To my astonishment, Wendell rapidly went into a complete Remission (blood and marrow became normal) and missed a Sunday on the pulpit for nearly two years. I had several other patients who were members of his church who reported that while he had always been a brilliant preacher his extraordinary sermons usually went right over their heads. However, since his diagnosis, the sermons had become more relevant and spoke right to their hearts. The church size had nearly doubled.

Wendell did not get very sick from either the leukemia or the treatment for a long time. He put up with a lot of hassle and lived under the weight of uncertainty and a dreadful diagnosis, but we seldom knew it. He looked good, had a full head of hair, and didn't physically suffer much. I never doubted his sincerity, but I wondered how it was going to play out when he got really sick and could see the tape at the finish line getting closer and closer. *I had seen a number of Christians claim their divine healing (which he did not) who crashed when it didn't play out as expected and the way they had scripted it for God. When it seemed God hadn't delivered, they started to question the reality of God and the validity of their faith.* I wondered how Wendell would handle the really sick days.

I found out. Wendell's leukemia disappeared for over a year before it slowly returned. Then it smoldered leaving him in an ever precarious situation with inadequate infection fighting and blood clotting cells. It caused him to crash repeatedly with high spiking fevers, bacteria in his blood stream, life threatening low blood pressures, and bleeding. *His outlook and demeanor never changed. He credited his certainty of God's plan for his life for his ability to live each day fully despite the uncertainty of his disease. Again I asked him where that certainty came from.*

*He said, "I learned to wait on the Lord, sometimes a long time, and he has never let me down."*

# TIME TO WRITE THE REST OF YOUR LIFE'S SCRIPT

The "never being let down" made sense, but I didn't quite grasp what Wendell meant by "learned to wait on the Lord" until my own life was on the line. *It seems that waiting is a litmus test for trust and a critical third part of any trust experiment with God.* Before we move on to that part of my trust experiment with God, take a few moments to review the key things presented in this first phase of trust experiments and what they mean to your current situation.

*Learning about Jesus may inspire you to believe, but only experiencing Him can inspire you to trust.*

*Do you know **about** Jesus or have you begun to **experience** Him? Write an example of how you have personally experienced Jesus.*
(Whoa! If someone had asked me to do that, I would have responded with "no way – don't like writing and don't have the

time." I would encourage you to try anyway. You'll be amazed at what comes to mind as you start putting pen to page. Try it.)

## Be a Scientist

*How did the analogy of being a scientist help you in your trust experiment with God?*

*Write about a time when you did your own trust experiment with God.*

## Expecting God to be God Leaves Him Room to Surprise You

*Record an event that has proved this to be true in your life.*

# A WINDRUNNER'S JOURNAL

*I invite you to reread every sentence above which is **bold** and in **italics.** Write it down, in your own words if you wish, to remember it, reflect on it, discuss it, or even memorize it.*

_____

_____

_____

_____

_____

_____

_____

_____

_____

_____

_____

_____

_____

_____

# CHAPTER 4

# THE TRUST EXPERIMENT: LETTING GO, GRABBING HOLD, AND HANGING ON

Trust experiments require three phases to move forward with God—much like crossing the ladder on a jungle gym. You have got to let go, grab on, and hold on over and over again to move forward.

*First, let go of or surrender your own agenda and its preconceived expectations, then grab onto His agenda without clear expectations, and finally hang on long enough to see it all play out.*

That doesn't always mean giving up on your own ideas. Yours and God's may be identical, but if they aren't, you have got to be willing to let go of yours to go with His. After all, He is God and you are not. He will know exactly what's going on in your heart and that is probably more important to Him than whatever is going on in the laboratory of your life. He cares about that, too, because you are the apple of His eye, His beloved child (Deuteronomy 32:10). Your happiness today matters to Him, but not as much as your happiness in eternity. Ultimately, we find ourselves facing something no one relishes: the idea of surrender which is inextricably tied to trust.

## The Trust Experiment - Phase 1
### *Letting Go: The Surrender Paradox*

I met a young couple who had married late in life and were in the early stages of discovering the wonders of what it meant to go through life together. His name was Willie, and hers was Donna and they were a delightful set of contrasts. She was large, he was small. She was a businesswoman with an MBA. He was carpenter who might have graduated from high school. She was neatly coiffed and he was scraggly. She could have just walked out of a board room and He could have just stepped off the fore-deck of an 18th-century schooner with a broad smile, scruffy blonde mustache and beard, unkempt hair, and dazzling blue eyes. When he wasn't working, he was dreaming. Her life had probably been one of discipline with achievement and his clearly had not. In fact, he had a pretty salty back story not to be told in polite company.

Sadly, he had incurable metastatic stomach cancer when we first met which we treated aggressively yielding great responses with durable remissions. They were able to go on with their life: Donna to the office daily and Willie to remodeling their kitchen between jobs that actually paid wages.

They were spiritual neophytes. Neither had been proselytized or "churchified." No religion had either blessed them or burned them. They simply had not given God more than a passing thought. To them, the Lord was unknowable simply because they had never been introduced. Jesus was just another historical figure along with Einstein and Churchill.

They were intrigued to learn who Jesus actually claims to be and even more curious to hear of His desire to be in a living conversational relationship with them. Not only a partner in their lives, but one who could shepherd them through the trauma they faced. At the thought of the heaven described in the Bible being real, they became fully engaged. I encouraged them to go discover who Jesus is for themselves and pointed them to the scriptures and several churches. Much to my surprise, that is exactly what they did. It was as if I had written a prescription and they went out and filled it.

They came back bubbling. It was as if Willie suddenly heard God call his name. He felt wrapped in the Lord's arms as if he had heard, "You are my beloved son." Something he had never heard from his own father. Loving acceptance, validation, encouragement, and a sense of place and safety had never been in the lexicon of his life until he met Jesus. Then something happened to Willie; it was as if the salt in his veins was exchanged for sugar. He became a new person and everyone noticed.

Neither Willie nor Donna had caring or trustworthy parents. Neither had privileged childhoods and neither had any sense of entitlement. So, meeting a God who was both loving and calling to them got the common "sign me up now" response. What was uncommon was that they did not stumble when they discovered that "sign-me-up-I'm-all-in" also meant surrender, the most difficult word in almost any language. The pride and self-centeredness that calls to most of us was not an obstacle for them nor was a gambit of bargaining for healing. They just opened their hearts and lives to divine guidance and waited with eyes wide open like children to see what happened.

Willie had never had a big brother or a mentor and his dad's advice wasn't worth much, so Willie was astonished to meet a God who would speak into his heart with both comfort and leadership.

*His response to the surrender challenge was, "Look, I'm gonna die soon and relinquish it all anyway. Why not give it all to God now and see where He takes me."*

Surrender is not easy for those with privileged upbringings or natural gifts of athleticism, intellect or beauty for whom their wellbeing is a matter of their merits rather than a blessing from above. For them, surrender can be nigh to impossible. Willie had never known the burden of such privileges, so it came easier.

*Surrender is also harder for men in general who have often spent their lives trying to develop self-sufficiency, establish their adequacy, and just plain prove they have what it takes! Willie had struggled with those issues, but even without them God's love affirmed he was capable enough.*

Surrender usually conjures up a picture of a beleaguered combatant, humbled before a victorious captor, the willing act of a defiant, unwilling heart. Surrender for Willie was much different. It started with an invitation from God rather than a demand. That led to an elective choice rather than a defiant capitulation. Surrender came after getting to know God, not in order to meet Him. With it a romance began rather than an imprisonment—a comfort and companionship rather than misery and loneliness. Willie knew he could renege on his choice and take any or all of his life back from God at any time, but never did.

Confession and contrition also came easy for Willie because they were his response to an invitation of a caring God rather than the demand of a red eyed irate father. Repentance didn't hurt when followed by a hug instead of a whip. I think he was so loved and accepted by Donna that it was easier for him to imagine the same and more from God. He no longer needed to manipulate circumstances to assure his control and security. Love and acceptance made control unnecessary so he could painlessly part with it. Surrender brought a kind of freedom he had never known and little expected.

I never saw any wickedness in Willie, but sensed there was some dicey history hidden somewhere—perhaps in his attic probably laced with shame—sort of like many of us. Worry and anxiety were probably there also, but after clearing his attic with Jesus, his freedom from them all was palpable. I didn't see a gritting of the teeth or a mustering up of determination to be good kind of change in him. Instead, a comfortable humility emerged as the tinge of inadequacy and the posture of apology receded. *A new liberty to just be himself emerged and he became a happier man—even though the death threat of cancer never changed.*

# DAY 1

# A WINDRUNNER'S JOURNAL

*I invite you to reread every sentence above which is **bold** and in **italics**. Write it down, in your own words if you wish, to remember it, reflect on it, discuss it, or even memorize it.*

_____

_____

_____

_____

_____

_____

_____

_____

_____

_____

_____

_____

## SURRENDER, THE PREREQUISITE OF TRUST

**"You need to surrender the way it has to be. If the only way you can be happy is when life turns out the way you imagined it, you are not going to be happy very often."[1]**

"Remembering that you are going to die is the best way I know to avoid the trap of thinking you have something to lose. You are already naked."[2]

Willie told me it was scarier to hold onto control without knowing for sure where he was going by himself than to surrender it all to trusting the Jesus he was just getting to know.

It seems our default setting at birth as part of our human nature is "do it my way." Eve certainly had it, teenagers fight for it, and powerful bosses and politicians abuse it. Many who decide to give their lives to Jesus are thinking, "Sure I would love His divine power and help in my life, so I will follow Him, as long as He is going my way and as long as I am calling the shots."

The core problem with the prideful "my way" is not that it is always wrong, but it rejects that God's way might be better and precludes trusting Him. Because He knows we are strong-willed and self-centered, God has given us decades to figure this out. If you might not have decades left, it might be worth doing some faster figuring.

The Dragon knows this about us, too, and exploits it. He adds an unforeseeable consequence to anyone's insistence on "my way" which is the lurking fear that it won't work and that we won't get our way. That produces anxiety, destroys peace, and begets sleepless nights, agitation, heart disease, and lousy relationships. The Dragon foresees it all and wins when it seduces us into holding fast to "my way."

*However, surrendering "my way" to "His way" frees us from the Dragon's ploys in this life and promises a good and certain future in the next. Still, many feel that gambit is just not worth it. Not knowing that God promises to give us life "abundantly," they hesitate to trust Him for fear He will wreck it. Yet if it is already wrecked, they look to Him for a quick fix.*

No matter what "it" is, He is willing to fix it, but only on His timetable, His way, and only as part of a whole package deal. Imagine if you drag your sorry overheating automobile into God's workshop asking Him to add some cold water to the radiator and fast. His response is most likely going to be, "Slowdown pal, I'll help you fix your car, but let's start by figuring out why it is overheating." You see, there are no shortcuts with God!

# Day 2

# A Windrunner's Journal

*I invite you to reread every sentence above which is **bold** and in **italics**. Write it down, in your own words if you wish, to remember it, reflect on it, discuss it, or even memorize it.*

_____

_____

_____

_____

_____

_____

_____

_____

_____

_____

_____

_____

## Surrender to Trust Brings Freedom

*What freedom could possibly come from surrendering your life to Jesus? Allegedly, it is freedom from an unrecognized prison and the burden of directing every decision or having to control every outcome, person or natural phenomena.*

Many respond, "I like control – it's no burden. What is this freedom anyway? If the walls of the me-in-control prison are real, they sure are invisible." Consequentially, escape is simply unimaginable to someone who never been on the outside. There is no better slave than the one who doesn't know he is a prisoner or ever dared to imagine what freedom might feel like.

Most of us have experienced the challenge of planning a day of activities with some combination of fun and work, and in the end felt trapped trying to make it all fit into the time allotted. As time evaporates, stress amps up. Anxiety rises. The timeframe of a day compels us to plan and to worry—just the opposite of trust and peace.

We do the same thing with our whole lives. We have things we need to do or ought to do, and ones we want to do before life comes to an end. Any uncertainty about when the end is going to come, particularly if it might come early, can cause extraordinary anxiety. As soon as we recognize the limitations of a timeframe, we feel like the freedom has been squeezed out of life. Our media driven agenda is threatened.

Ostensibly, we have two choices. We can speed up to accomplish our agenda and feel frenetic, or we can prune back our agenda and feel deprived. However, there is a third and better choice. Surrender our agenda to a better planner and then rest in peace that a good God is a good planner. Here is the bonus: *He promises to **always** provide enough time for what He has planned.*

## Insurgency, a Reaction to Surrender

*To even consider the possibility that Jesus is who He claims to be and that the transaction He offers is credible, is to enter into warfare with yourself. Expect a clever dragon inspired insurgent self to go to battle with any new thinking. Committing your life to the Lord does not end the war, it only marks the victory of the first battle. The self does not give up easily.*

Barack Obama spoke in a common idiom of counter-insurgency warfare when he addressed General McCrystal on the eve of attacking Marjah in Helmond Province of Afghanistan, "Do not clear and hold what you're not willing to build and transfer." This is apt advice for those on a journey with Jesus battling their own self-centeredness. It is not enough to confess and commit your life, if you're not willing to build a relationship with Christ and transfer authority to Him in region after region of your life.

In Afghanistan, the insurgents look like civilians who have always been there. Everyone is comfortable with their presence until they blow something up. Your enemy is every bit as homegrown and stealthy. It is hiding behind the virtuous self-will that gets you out of bed every morning and does every good and meaningful thing in your life. Whether you call the enemy the devil or just your own self-centered, self- aggrandizing, self-gratifying, and self-actualizing nature doesn't really matter. It is a natural part of us that lies in wait, a disguised insurgent called "self," eager to take back what was his: total independent control of your every decision. It is an opportunist who will take you out while you are on the road to freedom. Jesus will tell you where the IEDs are, but you have got to be listening and trusting what you hear in order to avoid them.

*Even so you will step on some. But stay engaged. "We grow spiritually much more by doing it wrong then by doing it right. That might just be the central message of how spiritual growth happens; yet nothing in us wants to believe it."[5]*

## GETTING REAL

*The best defense against insurgency is to get real with God.* That involves letting down the defenses of self-justification constructed over years and made impregnable for our own protection in every social arena. It means a willingness to be known for who we really are, which of course He already knows but is waiting for us to figure out. Such realness means abandoning

---

5

each façade of looking smart, looking good, looking successful, and abandoning our own so effective schemes of hiding and deceit. They don't work with God anyway, any more than they work for the three or thirteen-year-old with his parents. Just off load them like unnecessary baggage.

"The first requirement in a personal relationship with God is to be ourselves.

Off with the masks. Away with the pretenses."- Eugene Peterson[3]

*It doesn't mean you can't be smart, good looking or successful; you just need to understand that is not what matters to God or to most other "real" people either. It is only when you get real with yourself about who you are and what you feel, that you can get real with God. It is only when you are raw and real with God that you will hear and understand His raw and real answers. You are then set to do the same thing with your most intimate circle of spouse, family, and friends. As you let yourself be known, the comfort grows! His compassion for our circumstances will bring comfort but not permit us to rest in self-destructive wallowing. He will call us to rise out of it and to move forward with His direction.*

"God feels our pains, but He does not indulge our self-pity." – William Young[4]

The world and its churches are filled with incomplete Christians. Sometimes I think that must be the reason God gave us so many years to figure this out—a whole lifetime to become. We all know people who announced their decision to become something—say a musician. They start working at it so we call them musicians. However, some lose interest along the way and stop practicing and remain just mediocre musicians.

*The same happens to Christians. They started off walking toward Christ and may get close enough to follow Him for a while, but as their comfort and safety grow they start lagging further and further behind until they can hardly see Him. They may call themselves Christians, but it means very little. They never really got to know Jesus well enough to trust Him and want to spend time with Him.*

Over months and then years, I saw Willie and Donna explore faith and saw it become a major focus of their lives. It wasn't the usual "save my bacon God and I'll believe "gambit that so many cancer patients get into. Theirs was a fascinating journey of discovery that added a new dimension to their marriage and gave them a whole new perspective on his disease and their life. It shifted from being the only story they knew, to only a chapter in a much bigger and longer story they were discovering together.

Willie had become the magic in the life of a woman who was blessed with smarts rather than looks, and wisdom rather than charm, who had married late, and some might have thought married down, but they would have been wrong. Willie had made her so happy and her life so rich that I wondered how she would manage without him and what would become of her faith when Willie ultimately died.

After he did, she told me she was thankful and felt blessed to have had such a precious chapter of life with Willie. Her new-found faith was still an adventure and it dared her to think that she would see him again. When she did she would tell him about the richness of the rest of her life only made possible by their journey together with God through the land of cancer. Donna blew me away with her words, gave me a hug, and she was gone.

# Day 3

# A Windrunner's Journal

*I invite you to reread every sentence above which is **bold** and in **italics**. Write it down, in your own words if you wish, to remember it, reflect on it, discuss it, or even memorize it.*

_____

_____

_____

_____

_____

_____

_____

_____

_____

_____

_____

_____

_____

_____

_____

## The Trust Experiment – Phase Two
### *Grabbing On*

The second part of the trust experiment is discerning God's input and grabbing onto it, which means acting on it. The third part is hanging on long enough to see it play out. We humans are an impatient sort, prone to abandon quickly any endeavor that doesn't go the way we expect. The hanging on is the waiting that puts real trust into action. God loves to be trusted – rather like us who were made in His image!

## GOD AND BUYING CARS

It is exciting to read the reviews in *Road and Track* magazine about the hot characteristics of the new cars. Talking to the salesman builds on that, but it is reading the manual that tells you what the maker promises you can expect and count on. Even then you start the test drive out slow and that's how you should start with God.

Start with the small stuff, the everyday stuff, but get started. I used to keep God in the garage saving him for the big and desperate stuff. When that happened, I didn't really know how He worked nor what to expect. I really had no reason to have any confidence in Him so I could hardly ask boldly for His help and be confident that it would come. Instead, I would just keep on worrying and wondering.

*Start taking God for a test drive, find out what He will do, and remember God says, "My thoughts are not your thoughts, neither are your ways my ways" (Isaiah 55:8). Proverbs 3:5 reads, "Trust in the Lord with all your heart and lean not on your own understanding." You may need to look for answers in some unusual places. The risk is small for you. Give God a try. Find out who God really is.*

So, start with simple questions, not with desperate ones. Once one is desperate, it is hard to discern God's voice because other voices of fear, anxiety, and confusion are already clamoring about in your head. I am convinced God wants to be involved in the everyday small things of our lives—even things that seem too trivial to bother Him with.

One evening a group of friends shared their "trivial" prayer experiences. They described asking God to help them find a parking place, help remembering where the car keys were, help changing a grumpy attitude, help controlling wandering lustful eyes, patience to deal with a quarrelsome child, how to love a spouse better, what to do about aging parents, how to speak to a spouse about irksome habits or whether to speak at all, and help with all kinds of daily decisions.

One offered **"It was when I started getting God involved in the minutia of my life that I discovered how much anxiety provoking minutia there really was. Trusting Him to provide answers to all those little anxieties resulted in a peace I didn't know was possible."**

When asked what it takes to earn someone's trust, one patient responded, "A lot." When he hires someone, the amount he will trust a newbie depends first on their credentials, then on the stature of whoever recommended them, but the rest needs to be earned. God wants to earn ours and will if we let Him. There is nothing esoteric about that process.

*"All truth must be experienced personally before it is complete, before it is authentic."*
*– C. S. Lewis*

This is certainly true before one can stake their life on it. This is every bit as true with relationships as it is with scientific facts. We do it all instinctively and intentionally every day with new acquaintances, during courtship, while raising kids, on the sports field, and at Boot Camp. The curious thing is that so many people don't do it with God when there are so many opportunities.

*Find something each day to get God involved in, little, everyday quandaries and issues. Choose things that you don't have to act on immediately. The key words here are "have to."*

*Find issues that afford you the time to wait for God's answers and then wait for them.*

Over time it will become a habit because the answers are something worth waiting for. Over time you will discover yourself getting Him involved earlier and earlier to be sure there is enough time for His input before you have to decide on your own. Over time, He teaches us to wait longer and longer, not because He's playing with us, but because sometimes we are slow to catch on and sometimes the best outcome involves His working with other free-will people who are also slow. As more answers are recognized, confidence builds, anxiety leaves, and peace arrives.

# DAY 4

# A WINDRUNNER'S JOURNAL

*I invite you to reread every sentence above which is **bold** and in **italics**. Write it down, in your own words if you wish, to remember it, reflect on it, discuss it, or even memorize it.*

_____

_____

_____

_____

_____

_____

_____

_____

_____

_____

_____

_____

_____

_____

## The Trust Experiment: Phase Three
### *Holding On Means Waiting*

## THE HARD WAY TO LEARN – MY WAY

I was sitting on our cabin porch one August morning at sunrise reading Isaiah 40:28-31.

> *Do you not know? Have you not heard? The Lord is the everlasting God, the creator of the ends of the earth. He will not grow tired or weary, his understanding no one can fathom. He gives strength to the weary and He increases the power of the weak. Even youths grow tired and weary and young men stumble and fall; but those who **wait** upon the Lord will renew their strength. They will soar on wings like eagles; they will run and not grow weary, they will walk and not faint.*

I was weary from working too long and too hard, so renewing strength sounded pretty good, but I didn't get the waiting part. I even naively prayed, "What does this 'wait on the Lord' stuff really mean?" I get it now, but I didn't then. **Waiting is trust in action.** It is the physical manifestation of a heart and mind conviction. It is the proof that belief, faith, and trust are real. When we are waiting, it is the answer from the Lord that is all important to us, but it is what is going on in the heart of the waiter that is all important to God—the trust it takes.

How does one learn to wait and trust? It seems there is an easy way and a hard way. I sure learned the hard way. The words **"WAIT and TRUST"** were repeated three times, booming through the stillness of an Arctic evening like cymbals in my head—a startling answer to frantic prayers. Alone in a mountain meadow, I was so stunned when I heard it, I even took my eyes off the bear to look over my shoulder to see who was bellowing at me. No one!

I wondered, "Is that the Lord?"

I'd never heard Him out loud before, but He was the only one who could have heard my silent desperate, "Lord, take this bear away **now**! Lord, bring my son Bryson and our guides with their guns back **now**!"

On that August evening out in the wilderness, it felt like I was getting hit over the head with a 2x4 explanation as the Lord was saying, "Wait on Me means wait for Me to answer and trust that I will."

Finally, it makes sense. The asking for help part of prayer is pretty easy—although even that takes some practice—except when facing a grizzly. The waiting patiently for His answer is the hard part. It always has been. It requires me to actually trust Him in my heart and that really takes time and practice. Conversely, if my actions don't show that I am willing and able to wait for God to deliver on His promises, it does show visibly and experientially that I don't trust Him! Not good and pretty hypocritical for a guy who thinks he is a believer!

There are some things I know, and some things that just seemed to be true. I know there was a bear running after me. I know I heard a command to "wait and trust." I know an amazing peace came over me when I realized God was there even though He was out of sight, and the bear was still just fifteen feet away.

It was an eight-foot tall, golden brown, standing-on-its-hind-legs grizzly she-bear. No cubs were in sight, *yet*. It just stood there looking at me in a rather bewildered kind of way. The wind from behind her blew her scent to me, but none of mine to her. I looked pretty strange, nearly naked and dripping wet from my plunge in the arctic stream by camp. I had just managed to get on my shorts having pulled them over my pumping legs as I ran barefoot up the trail. Strangely, that made me feel a lot better until I realized that the bear, who couldn't see me running away at first, had heard me and was coming after me anyway.

*It seemed to me that the Lord protected me, but that He also took advantage of a scary situation when He had my full attention to teach me some practical truths:*

1) *Waiting = Trusting*
2) *Despite all my education, I'm still pretty dumb and clueless about some stuff.*
3) *Despite all my preparation and planning for contingencies including a possible bear encounter, alone is alone and I still need God.*

## 4) *I can trust God to deliver me, but in His own way and on His own timetable.*

I had met the bear face-to-face walking back into our camp au natural after a pre-dinner (mine not hers) glacial bath. Son Bryson and I had come to hunt Dahl sheep in the Yukon and had just ridden 100 miles from our float plane drop off to make camp in the Snake River Valley. It lay between towering mountain ranges right on the Arctic Circle in the midst of grizzly country. Months of training and research had not prepared me for all I had to learn.

First, it was that a calm "shoo bear" doesn't work well when the bear can't smell you and does not know what you are. Humans are rather rare at those latitudes. Then I discovered that rational backing up slowly is fine, but once you are behind a tree and can no longer see the bear, rationality departs quickly and terror gets your feet moving in a hurry. I also learned that running, even when you are out of sight, is a bad idea. Bears have keen senses. They have great hearing and can even feel the ground vibrate from running bare feet. Like all predators, they love to chase things that run. When animals that big gallop, it looks like lumbering, but in fact they move extraordinarily fast. A bear can run thirty-five mph and can out run a horse in the fifty-yard dash.

Then I learned that the Lord can put some pretty strange ideas in your head just when you need them the most. The next move in **my playbook** had been to drop-down, cover-up my neck and face, go limp, play dead, and wait for the bear to bat me around while hoping it will lose interest faster than I lost blood. Then a bizarre idea came to me: run back at the bear, jump up on a big rock, throw my hands in the air, and give a growling scream at it with all the vitriol and venom I could muster to pretend that I was the predator.

Much to my surprise, when I did it the bear stopped cold in its tracks within spitting distance. Then it stood up on its hind legs and just looked at me.

I don't know where the chutzpa to carry out such a crazy idea came from if not the Lord. I had never heard of such a thing, nor was I thinking clearly enough to recall it if I had. Now in retrospect, this idea seems as silly as when the Lord told Joshua to march the Israelites shouting and horn blowing around Jericho to fall the walls.

With my prayers, the bear did not fall down, but it did stop abruptly. Then it paced back and forth and eventually it walked away. I remember an emphatic, "Yes, Lord" as I lowered my arms, but then it turned back toward me. Up again went my arms, my prayers, and my shouting. The bruin rummaged through camp before it just lay down and stared at me. Then it charged again and stopped again, and for four hours it rambled back and forth, but never came any closer than fifteen feet, as if the Lord had drawn a line in the sand and instructed her not to cross it.

My suspicion is that the Lord was letting the bear do what free-will bears do while all along messing with its head, maybe even reasoning with it. At the same time, He was showing me that sometimes it takes a God who respects free will a little time to work things out, and if I want Him involved, I had darn well better learn to wait in order to give Him time to work in a way that respects the laws of His creation. Sure He could do it in an instant and sometimes He does, but He usually likes to reason with His creatures and to work within the natural laws of His creation.

Knowing that the invisible, but all-powerful, usually silent, but awesome God is present helps, but waiting on Him is hard even when He tells you that it is precisely what He requires. It can be an especially lonely business, unless you talk to Him continuously. Pray I did. It helped, but I'm a guy and I run out of words quickly.

Then I remembered what a terrified climbing partner on Mount Rainier had confided to me when she ran out of breath and words. Laurie just started saying the Lord's name—every step and another Jesus—climbing that mountain one step at a time. So I tried that, and I also felt His presence and peace.

By now it was 11:00 p.m. and the arctic sun was angling behind the shoulder of a mountain to the southwest; I was starting to freeze. Then a rather curious idea came to me, sing. How strange is that? What does a guy sing to a bear? But it wasn't about the bear and it didn't matter that I can't carry much of a tune. It was about singing hymns to God which is just another way of talking to Him out loud. It made Him seem closer and the peace that it brought was amazing. Singing those high school Young Life songs and the praise songs from church reminded me God is awesome, caring, present, good all the time, and very much involved in my life.

*Somehow singing out loud chased out all other thoughts and fears. When I stopped, it was as if there was a vacancy in my consciousness that opened up a place for fear to rush back in and fester. So, I kept on singing until well after dark and the disappearance of the bear. I suppose its departure was a testimony to how terrible I sound, or more likely to God's intervention.*

I'll never know why the Lord saved my bacon (literally) this time while in other times and other places people have perished. I do know God is in the business of teaching us about Himself and it seems this was a lesson for me I don't want to forget. Perhaps He might have coaxed the bear away sooner if I wasn't such a slow learner. I don't believe He inspired the bear to lick its chops and come after me, but I'm sure He allowed it to. When He had my attention, He started to teach. Are there any bears in your life? Does God have your attention? Would you like to turn toward Him now or wait for Him to get out the 2x4 or maybe something bigger?

Despite God's promise to Abram that his long barren and aged wife, Sarai, would bear a son whose descendants would outnumber the stars, they grew impatient. Years passed, so rather than waiting, they chose to help God out with a plan of their own. Abram would father a child through an Egyptian maidservant, Hagar. That union yielded Ishmael only to be upstaged later by God who enabled Sarah to birth Isaac. God delivered on His promise on His timetable, but after fifteen years! That is a long time, but God never gave us a timetable for waiting and trusting.

Ishmael and Isaac didn't get along then and their descendants don't now. Since the beginning of time untold consequences have come to those who cannot wait. The Bible is replete with their stories as are our own. Best we learn rather than suffer.

As for me, I have learned to pray and wait, and sometimes wait some more, and pray some more and wait some more, sometimes six months, sometimes five years. How terribly foreign this is, but how amazing to experience how the watchful waiting has allowed God the chance to work in events of my life – to change circumstances, open doors, close doors, change my heart or change the hearts of those around me. Perhaps one of the most profound experiences has been when He has changed my heart so completely that something previously terribly important no longer mattered; or another circumstance where I discovered I was completely wrong, yet the outcome was completely right. Even more amazing was the arrival of an entirely painless ability to apologize and move on—not generally an aptitude from my own playbook.

Equally astonishing is when God changes my wife's heart. She gets the credit for letting Him. As a gifted and wise counselor of couples and individuals (and me) with a soft, kind heart, she is usually right about most things. When she isn't and we go sideways, she can get pretty hot, a real "jumper and shouter" (her words not mine...but accurate). Even though a small woman, she can have a very big presence and when her heart changes it's a big deal.

*Learning to disengage, pray, and wait has been amazing for both of us. For me, this means zipping my lip and waiting, giving*

*God a chance to work in both of us. He does and hearts change.*
*We see things differently and with more grace. Thank God.*

## THE EASIER WAY

There is an easier way to learn to **wait and trust** God than my
way. Most people trying to know the Lord are doing their own
trust experiments already, at least subconsciously. Others tell me
it must be a conscious effort, daily and diligently.

If there is a single attribute that separates the Windrunners
from everyone else, even from most Christians, *it is their ability to
get God involved early even in small things and their ability to wait
for His answers.*

Throughout the waiting they are trusting an answer will come
in time and be good. The stumbling block for many of us is our definition of "in time," by which most of us really means "in my time."

I was no Windrunner when I sat on the porch asking the Lord,
"What is this wait business all about?" I would pray when I needed
God, listen hard for maybe thirty minutes, and then go off and
do the godliest thing I could imagine that fit in with my agenda. I
seldom allowed God enough time to give me His response tailored
to my specific circumstance, let alone enough time for Him to
work out the solution in the lives of the people and circumstances
surrounding me and my issue.

*Sometimes His best outcome involves changing the hearts,*
*attitudes, and actions of other freewill people (or bears) who can*

*be as slow and dense as I am. When I imagine how slow I can be, it helps me see why God needs time to move in other people including doctors.*

Anyone can know what to believe. They can even say what they believe. They can even preach what they believe. However, it is not until they act on what they believe that it becomes real. There are many circumstances in life in which God will participate given the chance. It seems we need to invite Him into our circumstances and wait for Him to reveal Himself in the outcome. In my experience, there is no more difficult situation in which to do this than when faced with our own possible death or that of one near and dear. God wants to be involved and He has both plans and promises just for you in just this moment.

**Trusting God puts *belief* into action.**

**Waiting on God is putting *trust* into action.**

**Waiting on God becomes the visible/experiential manifestation of trusting God.**

*Every day is about trusting God with more and more, and longer and longer until more becomes everything, and longer becomes forever.*

# Day 5

# A Windrunner's Journal

*I invite you to reread every sentence above which is **bold** and in **italics**. Write it down, in your own words if you wish, to remember it, reflect on it, discuss it, or even memorize it.*

_____

_____

_____

_____

_____

_____

_____

_____

_____

_____

_____

_____

_____

# Time to Write the Rest of Your Life's Script

If you're going to participate in His kingdom, you need to be able to trust His promises and be able to wait for His plans to reveal themselves day by day. That takes a lot of trust which has to be built through a myriad of trust experiments over time. So you had better get on with them PDQ. God gives us a lifetime to figure this out, but if you eat your vegetables now, you will get to have desert early—especially important if you might get called away from table early.

When you don't know what to do and urgency doesn't compel you to act in haste on your own, stand still and wait for the leading of the Spirit. As the gravity of the situation rises and time permits, wait until there is the convergence of the four ways God can speak to guide you and record what you discover:

- *Circumstances*
- *Impressions of the Spirit*
- *Passages from the Bible*
- *Godly wisdom from Christian counsel[6]*

# CHAPTER 5

# PROFILES IN TRUST

*"The proof of real faith is a changed life. A changed life that endures the ultimate hardship of facing death is worthy of attention."* - Unknown

*"You never know how much you believe anything until its truth or falsehood becomes a matter of life and death for you."* – C. S. Lewis[1]

*"You can say a rope is strong, but the moment you need to hang from it over the abyss is when you find out whether you really believe what you profess. Only real risk tests the reality of belief."* – C. S. Lewis

I don't think people were listening when Wendell spoke of his growing anticipation of what lay in store for him in Heaven. They saw a blessing and expected a cure, so many were caught off guard when he died. He never bothered to think about whether he would get or deserved divine healing. His focus was on what God had for him each day, always confident that more of everything lies beyond. Understandably, some who depended on him were more drawn to claiming his healing and seemed to struggle with God when death disappointed them.

Over the months, Wendell's words went right into my bloodstream and have been there ever since. Scripture came alive for me in him. I kicked my spiritual journey out of neutral, pulled my questions off the shelf, and started searching. I wanted to understand how God had entered this man's life and where this confidence and hope came from.

I started recognizing other patients who were living life like Wendell and began listening to and watching them closely. *They seemed to accept that God allows variability in this life which creates uncertainty so that we might wrestle with it, find Him, and the certainty of His plans that are behind it all.*

## BECKY - A WIN/WIN SITUATION

I remembered the year before I met Wendell when I had been so startled by the seemingly incongruous words of the mother of a patient who was actively dying. Her daughter, Becky, was a vivacious seventeen-year-old who had developed a painful swelling in one of her ribs which proved on biopsy to be a high grade Ewing's sarcoma, a rare kind of cancer which grows with lightning speed and is almost invariably fatal.

We all held our breath as we aggressively began the best chemotherapy we had albeit archaic by today's standards. Given perfectly, it is terribly toxic and in the way I gave it even more so. It put her in the hospital for weeks with a suppressed bone marrow, no infection fighting white blood cells, teeth chattering chills, spiking fevers, an ulcerated mouth, and a semiconscious delirium. I was despondent recognizing that the treatment I had designed was probably going to kill her before it had a chance to cure her.

Her mother kept a bedside vigil, ever sad but always calm and prayerful. On evening hospital rounds late one night, I remember walking down a lonely hospital corridor trying to find the words to tell Mom that Becky wasn't going to make it.

Sensing my anguish, *she* put her arm around *me* and spoke words of comfort and confidence, **"Becky is in the Lord's arms and He will take good care of her whether she gets to stay here with us or she leaves here with Him."**

I was stunned by her peaceful confidence and didn't understand what was going on until I saw Wendell who showed me. God was present and so was a kind of knowing and trust I had never seen! To my astonishment, Becky recovered from the chemotherapy and was cured of her sarcoma. She has gone on to get married and have a passel of kids, despite the repeated doses of chemotherapy which virtually always cause sterility. I don't know why God miraculously stepped in to alter biological natural history this time, nor why there are other times He does not. Maybe for Becky's sake, maybe because He has plans for her kids, maybe just to answer the fervent prayers of a trusting mother, maybe to affect my life, or maybe so I can tell this story to you. God knows.

## JIM – IN GOD'S HANDS

I'll never forget Jim. I had not known him long, but recognized right away that he knew Jesus. I didn't know how well or that I was about to find out. It was within a year that I joined a community of friends to gather around him to pray the night before his brain surgery. Six months of headaches had led to the discovery of a glioblastoma multiforme, the most aggressive of all brain cancers. While the neurosurgeon was capable and confident, we were all petrified, except Jim. There was something unmistakable in his demeanor. It wasn't a cavalier calm or a macho bravado, it was an abiding peace.

**"Look, I'm in God's hands, always have been, always will be, end of story."**

That evening he spent enjoying his friends and engaging in their lives, not focusing on his own. Within twelve hours, surgery was over and he never woke up, at least not to this life. I'm assured he is alive and well— just not with us. He knew something that we are still learning which made all the difference. I will never forget what I saw in the eyes of someone who placed all his trust in Jesus.

## CONNIE - THE TRUST GAP

Connie Jacobsen was one of my mentors long before he was surprised by cancer. He taught me about the Trust Gap—the distance between what we aspire to trust God for and the trust we put into practice. He taught me that because our lives are so full and fast paced, we seldom take the time, risk or effort to get God involved, and even less often recognize all the times He has gotten involved, even when not invited. Our ability to trust neither has a chance to be validated nor grow. Instead, the gap between the trust we profess and the trust we practice expands.

Connie pointed out that only regular practice in trusting God will shrink the gap and only then can you realize the power of what you say you believe. Belief is only a bunch of words about what you think. Trust is what we do with what we think. Trust is belief in action. However, it cannot be self-created or self-supplied; it can only be received and only if we return again and again offering up the unknowns of our lives with arms wide open to receive God's response. We need to join with the father in Mark 9:24, "I believe, help me overcome my unbelief." I want to trust, help me to do so. Just that invitation invites God's Holy Spirit to provide the power and wisdom to trust and the power and endurance to wait.

It does involve getting vulnerable with God. While it is flippantly easy to acknowledge that God knows everything about us, we so often fail to confess what we know inside are our weaknesses or inadequacies as if denying them will somehow obliterate them. Getting vulnerable with God is the first step toward experiencing His response: His loving understanding, forgiveness, acceptance, and assistance. It is also a huge step toward being able to be vulnerable with special people, critical in developing intimacy with them.

***God is not after perfection in our behavior and obedience or else He would have created automatons.***

***God desires a relationship.***

He created us perfectly able to communicate with Him as we cope with those parts of ourselves and this world that could be better. An automaton has no desires, no needs, and no reason to be in relationship with a creator. We do. Isolation hurts. Loneliness hurts. Not being accepted or loved hurts. ***People and things can assuage the hurts, but they are not dependable, whereas God is. A relationship built on knowledge and experiential trust closes the gap.***

## ROBERTA - FREEDOM FROM THE TYRANNY OF TOMORROW

Roberta had ovarian cancer back in the days when we only had Compazine to treat nausea and the best drug we had for ovarian cancer was the most nausea producing, Cis-Platin. The poor patients who endured that drug before we discovered today's miraculous anti-nausea medicines would vomit their socks off. Roberta was one of them and I was the agent of her misery.

She would sit in the exam room next to the sink waiting for me to come in and promptly vomit as soon as I entered. She was a bank president who chastised me for calling her at work because the sound of my voice induced such retching that it alarmed everyone in the bank. I remember hearing a strained voice sputtering, "Don't (retch) call (retch) me (retch) at work – ever!"

Supercharged with energy and passions, she confessed to me that "hurry" had always been like a demon for her. When cancer threatened her life, the need to accomplish everything in an ever shrinking envelope of time nearly crippled her. She was always dreaming about what tomorrow must or might look like which dictated what needed to be accomplished today. Having cancer, she felt driven worse than ever with no room for spontaneity, no room for conversations that didn't relate to tomorrows necessities, and certainly no room for God or any ideas He might have to interject.

***It was not until she decided to trust Jesus and His promises of provision, that she was able to escape the tyranny of tomorrow.***

Only when she released her plans for achievement in the future was she able to accept God's plans for her in the present. Paraphrasing her, "Only when I was able to completely trust God's provision for my life, however long it might be, was I freed from the tyranny of tomorrow. Every day became a good day no longer marred by anxiety over tomorrow."

"It was like stepping out of time; past failures no longer dragged me down or compelled me to perform. The here and now became like a sacrament and the choice to be present in it conveyed a special grace for both the past and the future." She went on, "The realization that God always provides enough time for whatever He has planned for you each day or conversely He never expects more of you than what is possible in the time available has lifted such a burden from my workaholic back."

# DAY 1

# A WINDRUNNER'S JOURNAL

*I invite you to reread every sentence above which is **bold** and in **italics**. Write it down, in your own words if you wish, to remember it, reflect on it, discuss it, or even memorize it.*

_____
_____
_____
_____
_____
_____
_____
_____
_____
_____
_____
_____
_____
_____

## WHAT YOU CANNOT SEE

At the beginning of our journey with Jesus...

*we are called to trust what we cannot see,*

*believe what we did not hear from His own lips,*

*and act entirely on secondhand, if not third, fourth or fifth hand information.*

*The journey is about converting hand-me-down information to first-hand evidence.*

***It is a circular journey that starts at the point of decision and gets ever bigger. In order to trust God, you need to know that He is real, that He loves you, and that He wants the best for you, but then you need to give Him a chance to show up and prove it. Every time you experience some of His love and goodness you become willing to risk trusting Him a little more.***

In a novel, *The Shack*,[4] the main character, Mackenzie, is in the midst of a horrific experience. He does not know if there is a God, but if there is, Mackenzie would be furious with Him for letting his daughter die.

Then God speaks to him, "The real flaw in your life, Mackenzie, is that you don't think that I am good. If you knew I was good and that everything – the means, the ends, and all the processes of individual lives, is covered by My goodness, then while you might not always understand what I'm doing, you would trust Me. But you don't!"

*Mackenzie had not had his eyes open wide enough over the years to see God's goodness in his own life or in the world around him. He had not risked trusting God in the circumstances where he could have experienced God's goodness, so without that he could not trust God in the midst of his horror when he really needed to.*

## TRUST STAIRCASE

One evening, a group of men gathered for fellowship and a harvest dinner of quail, pheasant, and elk. As Afterwards as we settled around the fire in the barn loft for our ritual cigar and Talisker, we wrestled with a question. Is there something Jesus says, which if you really believed it in your heart and down to your toes that would change your life dramatically and forever? These were men thirty to sixty-years old who have been around the block of life with the Lord for a few, if not many years. Silence settled like a blanket over us. Some eyes searched the eaves of the room, others the depths of the fire.

Then one seasoned by life's storms, but ostensibly one who had it altogether, said, "If I could really trust Jesus that His agenda for my life would be better than my own – and that it would be as much fun, I would give it all to Him instead of just saying I do. Then my life would change dramatically and I could live with a peace which I now only fleetingly grasp." When Brooke stopped speaking, heads all around the room were nodding knowingly.

Then another question was raised, "If that kind of trust lies at the top of a trust staircase, what is the next step for you? What is the next thing you want to trust Jesus with?" Another sage friend replied, "I've arrived at the place of trusting Jesus with my life. I don't worry about whether He will provide for me or even how long I will live, but I worry about my kids. There are so many unknowns ahead for them."

Then his wife, Rebecca, who, with my wife, Suzanne, had been serving our lucky group, called out from the kitchen in her sweet southern drawl, "Honey, you know He has got a plan for them, too. He's gonna provide for them just as well as for you."

Nodding, Mark continued, "My head knows that, but it hasn't reached my heart yet."

***"That's the trust step on the ladder I'm trying to climb, but in the middle of the night I know I'm not there yet."***

These guys look like a successful bunch. They do what they do well. Some are skilled tradesmen, some businessmen, and others in service. They all seem to be self-reliant, self-directed, ever bold, rugged individualists, and for the most part leaders, the kind of guys our culture admires. What makes them so capable and admirable is actually their reliance on direction from God. He is the source of the confidence the world sees in them and He is the source of the resilience that picks them up when they fall down. The world sees "a man's man," but that is only because underneath is a "God's man."

*That is also what the world sees when they get sick. I suspect they will join the Windrunners. It is not about what the world sees. That is secondary. It is about what is going on inside of them that only God sees that matters.*

# Day 2

# A Windrunner's Journal

*I invite you to reread every sentence above which is **bold** and in **italics**. Write it down, in your own words if you wish, to remember it, reflect on it, discuss it, or even memorize it.*

_____
_____
_____
_____
_____
_____
_____
_____
_____
_____
_____
_____
_____

## TRUST TESTED

> *In order to know what is in your heart.*
> (Deuteronomy 8:2)

God likes to be trusted and He has been known to hang folks out to dry for a spell both figuratively and literally when they do not trust Him. He invited the Israelites to trust Him when He commanded them to march into and occupy Canaan the first time. When, out of fear they declined, He sent them back into the desert for forty years until the entire non-trusting generation had died off.

It is easy to understand how they could be fearful of large and fortified opponents, but why didn't they have confidence in God? Why couldn't they trust Him to deliver on His promise? He had just performed innumerable miracles before their very eyes as Moses confronted Pharaoh: turning the Nile to blood, infesting the land with frogs, killing Egyptian firstborn sons while sparing the Hebrews, then parting the Red Sea, and providing the bread of heaven, Manna, fresh and new every morning, and quail aplenty for them to eat. After all that, they stood on the edge of the Promised Land, 600,000 strong, and behaved as if God didn't exist and couldn't be trusted. They must've been blind to every way He had blessed them or incredibly forgetful or awfully fearful or all three. Their blindness and forgetfulness is not a great example to follow.

*Was it that they had not been individually prayerfully involved having left it all to Moses?*
*Did they fail to see God's intervention for what it really was?*
*Were they just going along for the ride taking it all for granted?*
*Are we just the same?*

Forty years later when it came time for the Israelites to enter the Promised Land, Moses stood on the shores of the Jordan River and spoke to them, "Remember how the Lord your God led you all the way in the desert these forty years, **to humble you and test you in order to know what was in your heart,** whether or not you would keep His commands. He humbled you, causing you to hunger and then feeding you with Manna, which neither you nor your fathers had known, to teach you that man does not live on bread alone, but on every word that comes from the mouth of the Lord. Your clothes did not wear out and your feet did not swell during the forty years. **Know then in your heart that as a man disciplines his son, so the Lord your God disciplines you**. Observe the commands of the Lord your God walking in his ways and revering him" (Deuteronomy 8:2-16 emphasis added).

A big test came when it was time to cross the Jordan River into the Promised Land and confront the people already living in Canaan. The Lord spoke to them, "This is how you will know that the living God is among you and that he will certainly drive out before you the Canaanites.... See that the Ark of the Covenant of the Lord of all the earth will go into the Jordan ahead of you. And as soon and the priests carrying the ark of the Lord set foot in the Jordan, it's waters flowing downstream will be cut off and stand up in a heap" (Joshua 3:10-13).

It was spring and the river was in flood stage, so walking into the raging waters meant trusting that God would keep His promise lest they be swept away and drown. "As soon as the priests... Set foot in the Jordan, the waters from upstream stopped flowing" (Joshua 3:15-16), and the Israelites crossed over walking on dry land.

*The Lord required of them to take a risky step of faith and trust, and then He delivered on His promise.*

He requires the same of us. We are to take a step of risk and trust in the direction He proposes and then He will come alongside us and provide whatever is needed. There are many "Jordan Rivers" in our lives. The last, the coldest, and the deepest is death. It takes a lot of trust to walk into it, but when you do the Lord delivers on His heavenly promises.

Their testing didn't stop when they crossed the Jordan. Curiously, the Promised Land they entered was full of people in fortified cities. God instructed the Israelites to attack town after town and kill everyone. Why would He do it that way? Why not just give them an empty land and make it beautiful? I wonder if it was to provide God an ongoing opportunity to show His power, but hadn't He already done that? It also provided the Israelites an opportunity to show their obedience, but weren't there easier ways to do that? Perhaps, but this command was unique. It required them to risk their lives repeatedly in mortal combat against enemies that their spies had described as "stronger ... and of great size... so much so that we seemed like grasshoppers in our own eyes and we looked the same to them" (Numbers 13:33). Over months and years the Israelites were placed in a position of risking their lives which they could only do if they trusted that the Lord would deliver on His promises–and He did. Wow!

Teaching and testing! They seem to be a *common modus operandi* for the Lord. Life provides the opportunities for us to risk, trust, and wait for Him to deliver which is a litmus test for faith. There are enough opportunities in daily events for us to engage Him and experience Him enough to develop trust deep in our hearts and down to our toes, so "that He who has started a good work in (us) will carry it on to completion" (Philippians 1:6). Period! To do this requires humility for us to take the ultimate step to surrender our need to act immediately and in our own way. If we can, there are dividends.

"True humility is a healthy thing. The humble man accepts the truth about himself. He believes that in his fallen nature dwells no good thing. He acknowledges that apart from God he is nothing, has nothing, knows nothing and can do nothing. But this knowledge does not discourage him, for he knows also that in Christ he is somebody. *He knows that he is dearer to God than the apple of His eye and that he can do all things through Christ who strengthens him; that is, he can do all that lies within* *the will of God for him to do ....**When this belief becomes so much a part of man that it operates as a kind of unconscious reflex... the emphasis of his life shifts from self to Christ**, where it should* have been in the first place, and *he is thus set free* to serve his generation by the will of God without the thousand hindrances he knew before."[6] Uncertainty is gone. Fear is gone taking with it worry, dread, anxiety, and sleepless nights. In their place is divine purpose that feels so right!

Can't you just identify with God? Isn't it just like when we ask our kids to go along with our grand plan and they keep whining, "Why, why?" and we reply, "Just trust me on this one." Like them, we little realize that while we are doing our trust experiments testing out God, He is really testing us. Are we ready for His kingdom? Will we trust Him day by day and ultimately with our very lives? Proverbs 3:5 says it all, **"Trust in the Lord with all your heart and lean not on your own understanding; in all your ways acknowledge him, and he will make your paths straight."**

If you have trouble trusting, you are not alone. Even after years trying to get the message through to the Israelites, God was sending the same message through Jesus, who speaking to His disciples said, "I've told you all this so that trusting me, you will be unshakable and assured, deeply at peace" (John 16:33

---

6    Richard Rohr, *Falling Upward, A Spirituality for the Two Halves of Life,* Jossey-Bass. San Francisco, CA. 2011.

MSG). Jesus knew testing was coming and was preparing them for it. They had been at the Master's side, but their trust had not been tested yet.

Webster puts it that, "Trust is often instinctive, less reasoned than confidence." Jesus wanted His disciples to have both and He wants you to have both. Your time of testing will come. Initially, most of the disciples failed theirs and went into hiding. Will you? With Jesus' resurrection their confidence was reborn. How about you? None of us can answer that question any better than Peter until we have an experiential knowledge of Jesus' trustworthiness that can build the confidence. Our ability to wait is a measure of both.

Peter instinctively trusted Jesus enough to follow Him after their first meeting and after three years of experiences with Jesus, he was confident enough to proclaim Him the Christ—the Messiah. Then Jesus told them in the upper room, "In a day or so you are not going to see me, but then in another day or so you will see me...you will be full of joy...you'll no longer be full of questions" (John 16:16-24 MSG). But Peter's questions defeated his confidence. He would soon stagger in confusion as he watched what had been foretold play out and then deny Jesus three times. Peter's confidence could not overcome his questions. We, too, will never cease to have questions, but when real confidence arrives, we can cease needing to know the answers.

# A WINDRUNNER'S JOURNAL

*I invite you to reread every sentence above which is **bold** and in **italics.** Write it down, in your own words if you wish, to remember it, reflect on it, discuss it, or even memorize it.*

_____

_____

_____

_____

_____

_____

_____

_____

_____

_____

_____

_____

_____

# DOES GOD GET EXASPERATED WITH US?

Perhaps, but hundreds of years of recorded history with the Israelites suggests God has unfathomable patience. Although it seems that God can get ticked off and choose to let life discipline those deaf and blind to His words, the forgetful and fearful, and the stiff-necked and hardhearted. The evidence suggests it is all in a loving attempt to get through to them. So, if it feels like you have been toughing it out in the turmoil of life, you might be well advised to consider if there is something you are forgetting or need to figure out. If so, it might be wise to get on with it as He may have more desert time planned for you. He's not asking for performance: 3000 "Hail Mary" declarations or a donation to the church development fund. He wants your heart to change and that takes time, so you had best get on with it.

> *I have learned to be content whatever the circumstances. I know what it is to be in need, and I know what it is to have plenty. I have learned the secret of being content in any and every situation whether well fed or hungry, whether living in plenty or in want. I can do everything through him who gives me strength.* (Philippians 4:11-13)

How could Paul do it? What did he learn? What does this "give me strength" look like?

*I believe it looks like confidence which translates to courage and stamina and comes from pumping spiritual iron: trust experiments.*

## SEEING GOD IN ACTION

*It is only when we venture into the deep water and get in over our heads, beyond the security of our own skills and strengths that we can truly see God in action. When we have the faith to respond to His calling and venture into an area of our weakness, we give Him a chance to show His power and faithfulness.*

Steve Furtick tells a wonderful story about cajoling his five-year-old son Elijah to venture into deeper water as they played at the seashore. With a father's encouragement overcoming a child's temerity, before long, Elijah was standing chest deep facing incoming waves with his father at his back and his hands stretched above his head in his father's grasp, anxiety written all over his face. Steve tells the story, "Finally, the wave arrives. Elijah screams to make sure I'm in position. I assured him that I'm right behind him. And at the last moment, just before the water wipes him out, I jerk him up high enough that the water doesn't even spray his face." This story sounds a lot like my life and the heavenly Father I know.

Furtick goes on, "Elijah laughs uncontrollably. Then he proudly screams. 'I am a wave jumper! Let's jump another wave, daddy.' I didn't have the heart or feel the need to explain that technically daddy is the wave jumper and he is the hand holder. We all know daddy is doing the heavy lifting here... my son's assignment on Team Furtick is simple and minimal: to keep his hands reaching upward and trust that when the wave comes, I'll lift him high above it."[2]

*This is the essence of audacious faith. A picture of how our faith and God's faithfulness work together when we trust Him to do great things.*

This is not a call to do wild and crazy things of your own invention. This is an invitation to boldly respond to God's calling and His agenda. One must be certain it is His voice that beckons you into deeper water and not a cleverly disguised voice of the world. *The arrogant often venture out into the deep of their own desires, only to discover that God's provision and protection are not there and never were.*

God certainly calls us to use the gifts and strengths that we recognize we have. The challenge for us is discerning in just what way He intends them to be used. There are also other aptitudes we have that God knows about but we don't. We often consider them weaknesses or disabilities, yet when we step out into them in response to His nudging, we have a chance to really experience who He is and what He is up to and build trust.

*Some day we will see and understand the outworking of God's plan in our lives. How His loving guiding hands have brought us to where we are, and how He laughed and cried and cheered as we fumbled, suffered, and prevailed through it all. Until then, we must trust.*

# DAY 4

# A WINDRUNNER'S JOURNAL

*I invite you to reread every sentence above which is **bold** and in **italics**. Write it down, in your own words if you wish, to remember it, reflect on it, discuss it, or even memorize it.*

_____

_____

_____

_____

_____

_____

_____

_____

_____

_____

# Trust Grows When Evidence Is Remembered

Evidence is the accumulation of many, often small clues that must not be forgotten. Prayers for help or guidance that are unanswered, or not yet answered, or answered but not recognized tend to flood the forefront of our consciousness making it hard in a crisis to believe God is even there. That is when the evidence of God's past provision is your stronghold. When you are jangled and discombobulated by a new stress, past evidence is hard to remember, especially if you haven't practiced accumulating and reciting it.

***Counting your blessings is a wonderful way to do that.*** Every night when I lay my head on the pillow and again if I awaken during the night, I start counting my blessings instead of sheep. I review the good things of the day and of my whole life. I haven't had a Pollyanna sort of life. It's been good, but I'll bet I can match most anyone for misfortunes and mistakes. Despite those, there have been some things that were and are just "inexplicably good" and others where clearly God has been at work. Counting my blessings is like reviewing His movement in my life. It builds my confidence in Him and my readiness to run to Him in moments of need. It is a peaceful way to fall asleep and an optimistic way to start a new day. Try it.

Some keep up a prayer journal that they periodically review to remind themselves when prayers have been answered. My buddy Chris has started a pile of rocks where each family member adds a pebble or stone or even a boulder whenever a prayer is answered. It is readily visible whenever they leave the house to remind them with every coming and going of God's provision. Joshua did this (Joshua 4:4-9). After the Lord had stopped the Jordan to allow the Israelites to cross into the Promised Land and He told them he did it so, "You will know that the living God is among you and that he will certainly drive out before you the Canaanites, Hittites, and Jebusites." After they crossed over on dry land, Joshua appointed twelve men, one from each tribe to collect a stone from the middle of the riverbed. They put them down at their new camp in what is present day Israel to *remind* future generations of the Lord's provision—and they are still there.

***Remembering God's provision was a big deal then and it is today as well. Do whatever it takes to remember God's provision.***

God moves, often unnoticed, in the lives of the people He loves even without their asking. Many people look back and see a boatload of evidence, if they bother to look. Give it a try and remember to tell it to your kids, friends, and spouse. The more you recount it, the more accessible and powerful the evidence will be when the crunch times come and an encouragement to all.

# Where Is God When I Need Him?

## Find the Evidence

I don't know how I met Emily, but I remember the despair in her eyes when I did. She was only a teenager and her mom was a single parent who had cancer. Actually, it was her second cancer. Actually, it was a relapse of her second cancer and she needed a high risk surgery right then. Emily's questions came cascading out like a torrent, "Is there any hope? Where is God? Will my real, but six-month old faith, survive this? I lost my faith the first time Mom relapsed and I have just gotten it back. It is so precious. I don't want to lose it but this is so big, so hopeless. I have so many fears. Will Mom die? Will she suffer? What becomes of me if she is gone? What about money—she can't work and I don't have a job and I have school!"

*What can one say without it sounding trite even if true:* **"God is here. He does want to walk every step with you. He is good. He will provide."** These all sounded like just words until we started looking for evidence in her life. There were all kinds of "serendipitous coincidences" or special good fortunes that had happened. Thinking back on them made it clear to her that God had been present and was providing for her even on that very day. Some were random happenings; others were answers to prayer. Collecting it all produced substantial evidence that God had been there all along.

The lights went on! The furrowed brow relaxed and even a smile emerged. She concluded that it is likely, if not certain, that God would be with her in the future. In Emily's case, it was the accumulated evidence of God's provision that made worry unnecessary. It wasn't that the circumstances had changed, but that her confidence based upon solid personal evidence had.

*What if she hadn't bothered to examine her past for the evidence? What if she had never invited God in her life? What if she had never prayed and sought His provision and guidance? Then there would be no evidence—the stuff we humans need. God would still be there, still willing and wanting to be involved, but without evidence we, as humans, would be hesitant to believe or put much stock in the possibility of His provision. It is so easy for the probabilities we see to cover up the possibilities of what He can provide. For her, worry and anxiety would have remained right in the space now occupied by confidence and expectation.*

## HAMSTRINGING GOD

One of Emily's fears was wondering where she would live if her mom's surgery led to prolonged hospitalization. What would she do if her mom needed prolonged postoperative care at home that she could scarcely imagine doing by herself? They had an invitation from her uncle to come live with his family across the mountains for as long as necessary, but Emily had ruled that out because she loved her high school and needed her friends.

So we talked about hamstringing God by limiting Him to our own personal agenda. It doesn't work very well. "But I wouldn't like it," was her understandable reply. So I asked, "Is it possible that God could change your heart and that you might eventually like it? Are you willing to give Him a chance at your heart? After all, if it is His best idea there must be something good, perhaps even special or meaningful about it for you, too. Kind of an exciting idea, right?" The lights went on again. Her brows softened. *"Hamstringing God—hadn't thought about that. Okay, I'll give it a try, but I still can't see how it will work, but I suppose He can...."*

## Day 5

# A Windrunner's Journal

*I invite you to reread every sentence above which is **bold** and in **italics**. Write it down, in your own words if you wish, to remember it, reflect on it, discuss it, or even memorize it.*

_____

_____

_____

_____

_____

_____

_____

_____

_____

_____

_____

_____

_____

_____

# Time to Write the Rest of Your Life's Script

Only regular practice in trusting God will shrink the gap and only then can you realize the power of what you say you believe. Belief is only a bunch of words about what you think. Trust is what we do with what we think. Trust is belief in action. However, it cannot be self-created or self-supplied; it can only be received and only if we return again and again offering up the unknowns of our lives with arms wide open to receive God's response. We need to join with the father in Mark 9:24 and tell God, "I want to trust, help me to do so." Just that invitation invites God's Holy Spirit to provide the power and wisdom to trust and the power and endurance to wait.

*Will you pray that prayer today?*

In order to trust God, you need to know that He is real, and that He loves you, and that He wants the best for you, but you need to give Him a chance to show up and prove it.

*Will you do this today?*

*Record what you are trusting God with or the decision you have asked His guidance with and then*

> *watch and wait for Him to show up and prove His*
> *way is what's best for you.*

Many people look back and see a boatload of evidence, if they bother to look. Give it a try and remember to tell it to your kids, friends, and spouse. The more you recount it, the more accessible and powerful the evidence will be when the crunch times come.

> *Begin listing your own boatload of evidence today.*

> *How did this affect your level of trust in God?*

> *Who did you share it with and what was their response?*

# CHAPTER 6

# OBSTACLES TO TRUST

Brennan Manning, author of *Ruthless Trust* points out the three greatest obstacles to putting trust into action are amnesia, inertia, and mañana.[1]

I would add to that FEAR UNDERLIES THEM ALL.

Often we can't act with trust because we have forgotten what God has already done, or just out of sheer laziness (perhaps better called cowardice), or the absence of urgency allows procrastination. The alternative which is easier and quicker than recruiting God into an issue is to simply do it our own way; which we know may or may not work, and yet we are willing to climb into a small-life prison cell with bars of fear and worry rather than taking a risky adventure with God. *We little realize that fear steals the empowered life we could have one risk and day at a time. The easy "my way" takes away from the trust-life we are meant to have that is expansive and faith generating. When urgency arrives, forgotten blessings cannot power trust and unpracticed prayers cannot guide action.* Even if you reach for the Bible, what good will it be if you don't know what power lies inside or where to find it?

Another obstacle is our need for convincing proof and absolute clarity about who we are trusting and where He is leading us. We crave certainty and to know both the path and destination of our journey – and that it will be safe. We all crave assurance of God's presence and faithfulness, something tangible, like solid gold that we can hang onto. However, you must prospect to find gold and you must mine your past to find evidence of God in action or you can pan for the gold in prayer in the present. You must search for Him to find Him and you must know Him or you won't recognize Him when He shows up. *Odds are He has shown up repeatedly in your life already and was overlooked- maybe in a storm or a hurricane where His mercies were in disguise.*[2]

## PERVERTED TRUST

Brennan also cautions us about how trust can be perverted: "In presumption, we assign to God the task of doing for us what we should be doing ourselves." We expect, because He can, God will intervene directly and secretly in human affairs in just the way we desire. In all good things God wants to be involved with you, but He does not necessarily want to resolve them for you, *presto chango*, at your command as your minion. **God wants to be involved in processing your problem—a process that indeed often produces the very results you want, but it is really the results IN YOU that He wants.**

We are outcome oriented, while He is process oriented. He already knows the outcome, but He invites you to enter in so you can learn and so you can enjoy the process with an assurance that it will be good even if it takes expanding your understanding of what good can be.

*If your cancer resolves or your ailing marriage heals or your financial calamity escapes bankruptcy without getting to know God better and without gaining a better understanding of who you are and what life is all about, then you have wasted your cancer and your strife. God won't help you do that.*

# A Windrunner's Journal

*I invite you to reread every sentence above which is **bold** and in **italics**. Write it down, in your own words if you wish, to remember it, reflect on it, discuss it, or even memorize it.*

_____

_____

_____

_____

_____

_____

_____

_____

_____

_____

_____

_____

_____

_____

# BEWARE ANOTHER PERVERSION: THE AMERICAN PROSPERITY GOSPEL

This belief system holds that God grants health and wealth to those who have the right kind of faith. It sprang from a metaphysical tradition of "New Thought," attributing power to the human mind: positive thoughts yield positive circumstances and negative thoughts negative circumstances.[3] This thinking is foundational for the development of self-help psychology and when extrapolated into the spiritual realm, tantalizes anyone struggling to regain control of their life after a cancer diagnosis has absconded with it.

It tries to solve the riddle of undeserved human suffering and provide an answer to the universal question of the afflicted, "Why me?" In so doing it serves up layers of guilt and delusion: follow the rules and you will be blessed, follow them not and you are doomed believing it's your fault. Not Jesus' gospel. A tenet similar to that of some churches that have driven countless parishioners from their pews to swell the ranks of today's growing cadre of "post Christians."

*"The prosperity gospel offers an illusion of control right up to the very end. If the believer gets sick or dies, shame compounds the grief."[4] I know this is true as I have witnessed it repeatedly. In my experience it is a ploy of the dragon, an enticing, semi intellectual deception like all the rest. It defeats every*

*meaningful part of a Christ-centered Bell Lap with false faith and false expectations until it is too late to discover otherwise.*

## CHRIS - CANCER CHANGED HIS LIFE FOR THE BETTER FOR A WHILE

## A DIFFERENT GOSPEL BUT AN INCOMPLETE ONE

Chris was educated and eloquent, and he could read "the writing on the wall"—no denial there. When I met him, he was even reading the small print. He told me he had been stuck in an ever broadening miasma of desires and aspirations unable to escape an ever present contagion: the fear of failure that twisted and blighted his every relationship and reached into every corner of his life. It was like a creeping paralysis. Spontaneity had died and an amorphous anxiety had settled over him like a wet blanket. He quoted Solomon, "So I hated life, because the work that is done under the sun was grievous to me. All of it is meaningless, a chasing after the wind" (Ecclesiastes 3:22). Then he went on, "I got esophageal cancer. After the surgery they told me that there was no evidence of disease remaining, but I still only had a 15 percent chance of being around in five years. I knew I was toast."

"So I left my job. I went from making a lot of money to not making much. Sold my big house and bought a small one. My priorities changed, my marriage really improved, and I am so much happier. I actually have more of the kind of time I value most, but there is another kind of miasma creeping in: I don't know what's coming. I am afraid of the unknown! Chemotherapy doesn't offer much and it's only a band aid anyway. I am beginning to bleed already and I can't even see the wound." Then he quoted a smattering of Ecclesiastes 6:12-14, perhaps imperfectly, but perfectly reflecting his outlook on life: "Who knows what is good for a man in life during the few and meaningless days he passes through like a shadow? Who can tell him what will happen under the sun after he is gone? God has set eternity in the hearts of men; yet they cannot fathom what God has done from beginning to end. It is all meaningless, like chasing after the wind!"

*He had no hope! His script had come to an end. He had finally tasted a better life, but the soggy blanket of despair was settling over him again. I wish he could have met Sally, or Karina, or Dave, Chuck, Connie, Al or Doris or so many of the Windrunners who knew the whole gospel. They had learned to trust Jesus and they had discovered something else as well— how to receive and practice hope.*

# A WINDRUNNER'S JOURNAL

*I invite you to reread every sentence above which is **bold** and in **italics**. Write it down, in your own words if you wish, to remember it, reflect on it, discuss it, or even memorize it. This short chapter only has two days for reflection. Use the other three days to do "Time to Write the Rest of Your Life's Script."*

_____

_____

_____

_____

_____

_____

_____

_____

_____

_____

# Time to Write the Rest of Your Life's Script

**Read the quote again: Brennan Manning, author of *Ruthless Trust* points out the three greatest obstacles to putting trust into action are amnesia, inertia, and mañana.[1] I would add to that fear.**

We crave certainty and to know both the path and destination of our journey and that it will be safe. We all crave assurance of God's presence and faithfulness, something tangible, like solid gold that we can hang onto. However, you must prospect to find gold and you must mine your past to find evidence of God in action or you can pan for the gold in prayer in the present. You must search for Him to find Him and you must know Him or you won't recognize Him when He shows up. Odds are He has shown up repeatedly in your life already and was overlooked- maybe in a storm or a hurricane where His mercies were in disguise.

How are you dealing with each of the obstacles to putting your trust in God into action that were discussed in this chapter?

>**Amnesia:** List the ways God has proven you can trust Him in the past.

**Inertia:** Get involved in the process. Don't expect God to do everything. List what you believe God would have you begin doing.

**Mañana:** Get to know God now so when the storms come in the future, you already have a relationship with Him. Begin to spend time with God every day. Record insights He reveals to you from reading His Word, the Bible.

**Fear:** Look up scriptures that have to do with dealing with fear. What does God have to say about allowing fear to overtake your life?

# CHAPTER 7

# CULTIVATING HOPE

What a treat it was to know Sallie. She was in her early thirties with incurable metastatic breast cancer when she walked into the cancer center with her husband, David. She was cute and he was ruggedly handsome, both totally committed to one another and to their son, Caleb. Hers was a totally unfair situation, too young, too innocent, and too angelic. Yet, she endured her chemotherapy without complaint and when she finished vomiting, the gentle smile would return along with her clever wit, "That was not fun, sort of like scrubbing floors: you gotta get it done before the party." There was something that kept her going with an effervescence that chemo could not stifle, and *joie de vivre* that the certainty of death could not quash.

Her remissions came and went over the years, but her spirits never wavered. When sadness came, she processed it, and gave it its place. Then she kept it there and out of the rest of her life. She told me that she had too much living to engage in than to let sadness get more than its due. When she couldn't downhill ski, they switched to snowmobiling. When she couldn't water ski, she drove the boat. When she couldn't play volleyball, she sat on the sidelines and cheered. Her life got smaller, but her heart didn't! Life was not about her it was about other people, the ones she loved and there were many.

Only a peace that surpassed all my understanding enabled such a life as hers. She told me about the ladder of her trust experiments (my words not hers) for that series of trials in her life in which she had chosen to trust Jesus, every rung a little higher, a little riskier, and every answer a little more profound—sometimes startling so, but always worthy of the trust. The peace that came didn't inspire her; it enabled her. It was hope that inspired her; it positively energized her.

***Those who abandon hope perish***. That was seen time and again in concentration camps and was an indicator of survival independent of nutrition or illness. I have seen it on the cancer wards time and again – and independent of the amount of cancer or organ function. "Those whose expectations of life are not met can give up. Survival depends upon discovering what life expects of us and in so doing find meaning."[1]

Chapter 5 in *The Bell Lap & The Dragon Behind the Door* extols the importance of developing a whole portfolio of hopes. But how does one do that when living in the shadow of possible death where the only ray of saving light is a tenuous, fragile, and singular hope for survival? C.S. Lewis described his experience living in that shadow in *A Grief Observed*.[2] He had been a devoted bachelor until he met Joy Davidman; she rocked his world, redefined it, and recreated it. Though Joy had breast cancer when they met, they "feasted on love; every mode of it – solemn and merry, romantic and realistic, sometimes as dramatic as a thunderstorm, sometimes as comfortable and unemphatic as putting on soft slippers."[2] They knew many hopes and most passionately, yet even when some of them failed, their enduring hope in Christ gave them the freedom and peace to experience joy. "It is incredible how much happiness, even how much gaiety we sometimes had together after all hope for survival was gone. How long, how tranquilly, how nourishingly we talked together that last night!"

## MYSTERY

Hope is a mysterious thing. Webster defines it as wistful thinking, but it is not the same as optimism. Optimism/pessimism are matters of optics, how you see something which depends on your mood which can be fickle or fabricated, vulnerable to unrelated irrelevancies, even an undigested fried oyster. The world does not really know what hope is or where to find it. Is it really any more than fantasy? Do you manufacture it or receive it? If received, is it of any more value than the trustworthiness of the giver?

*Biblical hope is "confident expectation." We know God cre-ated it, yet it is we who must discover it. He has given us an imagination and with it He inspires our hope, but even that can be little more than a vision until we live it forward—until we live into it; then it becomes real.*

I have watched many patients as they have sorted through a whole menagerie of hopes in search of one to sustain them, e.g., bizarre diets, mega vitamins, acupuncture, all kinds of enemas, and potions dreamed up by quacks of every description, spas, gurus, even chemotherapy. Some proved fraudulent and were painfully discarded, so search for a new hope would begin again. All had seemed so precious for a while, but too often proved disappointing. They weren't totally worthless, but they weren't worth much. As one puts less hope (hopes less) on them, a door may open to a divine hope previously unconsidered and only then discover how indispensable it can be. Perhaps that is why the Lord lets us get to the end of our rope and the end of ourselves.

It is okay to hold on to every hope you've got irrespective of its source just so that your God-given ability to hope can sustain you in the short run. However, recognize that your hoping may only be wishing. Indeed, it may be wishing for some things you already think are impossible and to which you already know, had you better sense, you would not commit your time, money or life. So, start prioritizing your hopes to find the one that won't disappoint. Day by day shuffle them, adding some, abandoning others. Having all kinds is okay as long as one of them is solid gold, independent of your biology or doctors and it is on the top of your list.

Sallie told me *"The only hope I have never seen fail grows out of a close relationship with Jesus."* Indeed, it is the very byproduct of that relationship. When you have it you can enjoy holding onto the others, but lightly—no longer desperately. When you are certain of Jesus you can live in peace despite the uncertainties of all the rest. Take that risk. The only alternative is lazy do-nothingness which leads to despair. So, it's your choice.

Another word for certainty is faith and together they leave no room for fear; where there is no fear, there is no anxiety. Building a relationship with Jesus to the point of certainty takes practice. It *takes practice to remember His promises and practice* to trust them. "They are the reality that is being constructed, but not yet visible."[3] At the beginning, faith in Jesus is small and the hope it generates is small, but with practice they grow together.

An overnight total commitment to become a runner doesn't make you fast and strong overnight. It gets you on the track every day where strength can grow. Some mistakenly surmise that a total, desperate commitment to Christ will give them access to all of God's power and hope, which it would if only they knew what is was and how to access it. That takes learning and practice. It is sort of like electricity. Your house can be wired, but you will remain in the dark until you learn how to plug into it.

Plugging in though takes an incentive. As Chesterton cautioned, *"As long as matters are really hopeful, hope is mere flattery or platitude. It is only when everything is hopeless that hope begins to be a strength at all. Like all the Christian virtues, it is as unreasonable as it is indispensable."*[3] **Unlike all the other tear-you-down feelings cancer** can contrive, this Jesus hope can build you up.

# DAY 1

# A WINDRUNNER'S JOURNAL

*I invite you to reread every sentence above which is **bold** and in **italics**. Write it down, in your own words if you wish, to remember it, reflect on it, discuss it, or even memorize it.*

_____
_____
_____
_____
_____
_____
_____
_____
_____
_____
_____
_____
_____
_____

## MAKING COMMITMENT

***Commitment begins spiritual transformation***. It is like beginning workouts in the gym that transform muscles. Even when they grow strong, it doesn't mean those muscles know how to play tennis, but they will be ready. Reading a book will help, but one has to get out on the court to learn the strokes. The forehand of faith is to trust. Each new challenge or tribulation in life is another ball coming across the net to try out your trust on. If you apply trust in God correctly, the ball will go into the court on the other side instead of long, short or wide. Only with swinging away will you figure out how it works. In that sense we can look forward to trials and tribulations as just one more opportunity for a workout with Jesus, and the better our game of life will get. It looks to me like those players at Wimbledon are having more fun on the court than we are. I suspect it is the good coaches and lots of practice. So as life keeps coming at you, if you put in the time with Jesus you will probably hit more winners and smile more while you are at it.

## NOT ALWAYS EASY

Sallie's wisdom was clever, raw, and real. ***"You know hope is buying into what you believe and it isn't always easy – not when you are sicker that squat and puking your guts out. Sure it is easy in happy-snappy land when you are healthy and singing*** *in the choir, but not where I'm at. When hope gets hard, I have to stay on fire and equip myself - be strong in the Word. I need to take up the 'Sword of the Spirit which is the Word of God' (Ephesians 6). I've gotta remember His promises in order to hang onto them"* (see Ammunition – Appendix 1).

## BEWARE

Hope can be tricky because it is so easily counterfeited. Oncologists sell it all the time to avoid having to talk about the hard issues. Friends proffer it to cheer you up and to protect themselves from having to deal with raw feelings, and we dream it up in a nano-second for all the same reasons. *However, counterfeit hope does not lead to peace that lasts or to real peace at all. It is the other way around. Real peace and real hope expose and protect against the phony stuff.*

> *Beware of the hope prescribed by a physician who has run out of good treatment options. Our teaching is to always offer something. One of the brightest cancer researchers, president of the American Society of Clinical Oncology, the most prominent research organizations in the world put this way: "We must always give them hope in order for them to live- never hospice." In other words, "never stop treating with new*

*medicines." He did not know Jesus and had no*
*other hope to offer.*

Fraudulent hope is only a convenient protective veneer against pain, a veneer that gets pretty thin when death is in the equation. The Dragon is pretty quick to point that out and exploit it. When it does, phony peace evaporates; fear raises its head sending people scrambling for new hopes to get their peace back. Some just give up trying as a wave of depression washes over them and the pall of the dragon's undertow sucks them down.

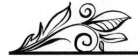

*"In order to be prepared to hope in what*
*does not deceive, we must first lose hope in*
*everything that does deceive."*
— **Georges Bernanos**

## Is Divine Hope Itself a Fraud?

Some assert that the happenings which occur outside our understanding do so without God's involvement simply as a matter of chance. Such assertion denies that God is almighty, the Alpha and the Omega, the creator of all things, omniscient, and omnipresent. I cannot do that; there is something bigger going on. God has not created suffering at all, nor permitted it just for the sake of suffering. He hates it and mourns it with us, yet He allows it. There is a reason, but is it is a mystery and it must be important. The consequence of the fall of man and our sin is only a pat answer.

*We are not meant to know more or He would have told us, but we are meant to engage Him fully in order to fully enable the outworking of His purposes in our lives.* There must be no other way for Him to accomplish such a goal in each of us or the loving God we know Him to be would have done it; just as there was no other way for God to reconcile all people to Himself except through the suffering and death of Jesus. So, it must be for us as we confront risk, suffering, and death.

*To know only God's good words is a distinct disadvantage if you haven't experienced God answering prayers in surprisingly and unexpectedly good ways, too. Only when you have let God surprise you can you really rest in the hope of His big surprise at Heaven's Gate. Risk letting Him surprise you soon.*

# Day 2

# A Windrunner's Journal

*I invite you to reread every sentence above which is **bold** and in **italics.** Write it down, in your own words if you wish, to remember it, reflect on it, discuss it, or even memorize it.*

_____

_____

_____

_____

_____

_____

_____

_____

_____

_____

_____

_____

## FINDING CONFIDENCE

I remember well during my faith journey when I came upon the word *confidence*. I immediately recognized that despite all the head knowledge I had from reading the Bible, listening to sermons and praying now and then, that I still didn't have confidence. In that moment, I realized the lack of it was what separated me and so many others from Bell Lap Windrunners who ran with peace and purpose, and yes, even joy. Abundant palpable joy! Not because running was easy; not because they were more capable; not because they were more blessed, but because they were less burdened by fear because of a confidence they had learned and earned.

I realized that even though I was not dying, such confidence was precisely what I longed for. I wanted it right then and I set out to find it. I wondered how could I get to that place called peace? What would it take? Was it even possible? Would I know when it arrived?

*The answer is that it is possible, and I did recognize it. The path was paved with countless conversations and trust experiments with God.*

It started with a lot of listening to my life and looking for the times God had showed up. However, the when, where, and why were not immediately obvious. My own past was readily available for study and more revealing than I initially imagined. Reflecting on it provided insights. With the insights, came contrition.

With contrition, came healing: a new found feeling of being forgiven, accepted, and loved. **I hadn't really recognized those as missing until they arrived. Sort of like the aborigine who doesn't miss having ice cream because he has never tasted it, but one mouthful later wants more and wonders where has it been all his life.**

With healing, came a new, less burdened, freer, and happier me, and a peace despite many persistent unknowns.

With all of that came a confident hope in Jesus that will extend beyond my last breath; it takes the anxiety out of all my other hopes: the hope that the metal in my back will hold, that my coronary arteries will stay open, that calamity will not befall my children and grandchildren, and the hope their educations will lead to meaningful lives with real and rewarding relationships. I find myself freer to hope for many things, but to hold them lightly and to not need them to play out my way. God has a bigger plan than mine. Perhaps it includes all those things or not, but I am certain it will be good. That is huge for me! There is something bigger going on here.

To some it would seem that God's promises for us in Heaven are utterly fanciful, something out of childhood fairytales. God's promises must have seemed like that to Abram when God promised him that his barren wife Sarah, age ninety, would bear him a son and that his descendants would be as numerous as the stars. Indeed, they did. So absurd that Abram fell to the ground and laughed. Genesis17:17 says, "Yet he did not waver through unbelief regarding the promise of God, but was strengthened in his faith and gave glory to God, being fully persuaded that God had the power to do what he had promised." Romans 4:20 tells us, "This is why it was credited to him as righteousness." How great is that! "Against all hope, Abraham, in hope, believed" (Romans 4:18). He did this when his body was 100 years old and "as good as dead."

*We are not only invigorated and comforted by accepting the hope that God's promises offered us both in this life and in Heaven beyond are real, but we are credited with righteousness (made right before God) by so doing and believing. Now there is a legacy worth passing on. One doesn't need to be wealthy, smart, strong or beautiful to do it.*

## HOPING FOR HEAVEN

William Stringfellow describes well the kind of hope that Sallie had: "*Hope is reliance upon grace in the face of death: the issue is that of receiving life as a gift, not as a reward and not as a punishment; hope is living constantly, patiently, expectantly, resiliently, joyously, in the efficacy of the word of God.*"[11] Sallie did.

Everyone around Sallie knew that it was Jesus who sustained her and that He often used David as His hands and feet, voice and arms. Together they never preached their faith, they didn't have to! Their life together spoke volumes. She was only thirty-eight when she died, but there were more than a few at her memorial service who envied the richness of her short life. They knew exactly where it came from and she had told them exactly where she was going. She would hum the song, *Spirit in the Sky*, and, if you didn't catch on, she would add the words:

> *When I die and they lay me to rest*
> *Gonna go to the place that's the best*
> *When they lay me down to die*
> *Goin' up to the Spirit in the sky.*

> Chorus:
> *Goin' on up to the spirit in the sky (spirit in the sky)*
> *That's where I'm gonna go when I die (when I die)*
> *Prepare yourself; you know it's a must*
> *Gotta have a friend in Jesus*
> *So you know that when you die*
> *He's gonna recommend you to the Spirit in the sky.*[6]

When such a wonderful mother dies, one wonders how the spouse and kids can survive the loss, but hers have. It is clear that the One who sustained her and made her the radiant person that she was, now sustains them. She passed the baton well, and David helped; he continues to remind Caleb of her words. Mom is still alive and is as indelible now in the memory of her words, as she is in Heaven where she is watching and waiting for them. Caleb was too old for bedtime story books, but children of all ages are always eager for a good story. She told him all about where she was going and how they would someday reunite, so day by day, night by night, together they let their anticipation grow.

When she died, she left all a parting poem to choreograph our feelings:

> *Don't grieve for me for now I'm free*
> *I'm following the path God lined up for me*
> *I took His hand when I heard Him call,*
> *I turned my back and left it all.*[8]

# DAY 3

# A WINDRUNNER'S JOURNAL

*I invite you to reread every sentence above which is **bold** and in **italics**. Write it down, in your own words if you wish, to remember it, reflect on it, discuss it, or even memorize it.*

_____

_____

_____

_____

_____

_____

_____

_____

_____

_____

_____

_____

_____

## HOPE BUILDS FAITH

Social scientists have shown that optimism (irrespective of its source) confers a survival advantage by helping people cope with adversity.[7] Hope in Heaven should fill our thoughts not only because it's fun to think about such wonderful prospects, but because it builds faith, enables loving service, and creates power to live for Christ each day in spite of every kind of hardship. Paul reminds us in Colossians 1:5, "The faith and love that spring from the hope that is stored up for you in Heaven." We can rejoice that we have a covenant God who keeps His promises even while we don't understand it all.

*Memorize and recite God's promises. Let them be the reveille that opens your eyes each morning and the reverie that closes them each night.*

"If you imagine everything will turn out the way Christ promises, you have every reason to be happy all the time provided you walk the path he calls you to."[9]

The challenge with God's many promises is to decide which one to focus on. Living teaches us to focus our hopes further and further ahead. As little children, we could scarcely focus beyond a promised ice cream cone after dinner. As grade schoolers, maybe we could focus out a week or two toward the promise of Christmas, as high schoolers maybe a few years until a job or marriage. By the time we are adults, we can look out a decade or three for the promise of retirement. Our capacity grows. Jesus invites our hopes to extend to a promised eternity, but we often don't pay attention until we need it.

The hope of such promises inspire and condition our experiences and behavior. How far do yours reach? You don't have to give up dreams of ice cream to focus your hopes on eternity, but when you do you can stop worrying about whether the ice cream will run out!

There are little promises and big promises, little hopes and big hopes. Don't confuse them. There is more ice cream in heaven than you can ever imagine.

## DAVE - AMMUNITION

We had spent twenty-five years of before work Thursday mornings sharing life and exploring God's Word together with a group of men, and just about that many chasing wild game in the mountains. One morning I returned from a predawn scouting hike to find Dave by the fire, coffee on and biscuits in the skillet. He was moving a little slow having just completed six months of prostate cancer chemotherapy, but his gentle rugged smile was as broad as ever. He took a cup of "joe" and moved off to one side and sat down to watch the sunrise play off the cliffs across the river. He pulled out some 3x5 cards from a pocket and began thumbing through them. Later when I asked what he was doing he replied, ***"You have to practice hope every day and these help."***
Then he showed me the flash cards he had made collating God's promises from all over the Bible. He would pull them out

like ammunition to chase away the Dragon, the feelings of doubt, confusion or depression. Sometimes he would pull them out just to "practice hope" and to reaffirm who Jesus is and Jesus' love for him. He carried them wherever he went knowing that with them he was always prepared for any misgiving. Now I have patients who collate them on their smart phones or call up one of several scripture apps.

> *The Lord is my light and salvation—whom shall I fear? The Lord is the stronghold of my life—of whom shall I be afraid? One thing I asked from the Lord, this only do I seek: that I may dwell in the house of the Lord all the days of my life, to gaze on the beauty of the Lord and to seek him in his temple.*
> (Psalm 27:1-4)

**Revisiting such verses fosters hopes and builds expectations, shifts them away from our fragile selves to our mighty God, displaces our trust from the doctor's agenda to God's where it belongs and is most secure.**

Many have followed his example, often using a smart phone or computer and found packing such weaponry was empowering. It is a great idea for any of us. I have collated in Appendix 1 "Ammunition" a list of the scriptures that Dave, Gale, Connie and others have found particularly helpful.

# Day 4

# A Windrunner's Journal

*I invite you to reread every sentence above which is **bold** and in **italics**. Write it down, in your own words if you wish, to remember it, reflect on it, discuss it, or even memorize it.*

_____

_____

_____

_____

_____

_____

_____

_____

_____

_____

_____

_____

# GALE - PRACTICING HOPE

Another way to practice hope and grow your confidence in God's promises is to get directly and personally involved in His work in your community and in the world. Many ask the Lord to bless the projects they dream up. That's fine, but there may be a quicker and better way to experience a hope inspiring blessing. "Get involved with what God is already doing. It is already blessed!"[9] You no longer have to wonder whether God will show up on your bandwagon if you are on His.

When you practice putting your hope into action by serving God's people, you will see Him keeping His promises and your hope will grow. There are hurting people everywhere, maybe in your own family, certainly in your community and definitely all around the world. Find them and find a way to care for them. Get involved. You will be blessed and your hope will grow.

*Then the King will say to those on His right, come, you were blessed by my father; take your inheritance, the kingdom prepared for you since the creation of the world. For I was hungry and you gave me something to eat, I was thirsty and you gave me something to drink, I was a stranger and you invited me in, I needed clothes and you clothed me, I was sick and you looked after me, I was in prison and you came to visit me. Then the righteous will ask him, Lord, when did we see you hungry and feed you?*

*When did we see a stranger and invite you in or needing clothes and clothe you? When did we see you sick or in prison and go to visit you? The King will reply, I tell you the truth, whatever you did for one of the least of these brothers of mine, you did for me.* (Matthew 25:34–40)

I met Gale when she was in college working with high school kids in Young Life and reconnected with her when she came to work in the cancer center. We lamented our loss when she married David, learned Arabic, and departed for Lebanon to introduce Jesus to Moslems. A blue-eyed, fair skinned, strawberry blond she probably got the melanoma on her scalp from the harsh Middle Eastern sun exposure where she lived and ministered with her David just a few miles north of the Israeli border. Figuring out how to deal with the biologic impact of her cancer was hard enough, but how and where to live with the uncertain length of her life was worse. Should she stay home in the relative safety of the United States near family and near the finest medical care in the world or return to all the uncertainties of the Middle East? Much prayer was in order and the answer emerged, not immediately, not easily but with profound clarity and peace.

The trust she had in Jesus' calling was bigger than either melanoma or Hezbollah. She took treatment but she chose to live in Lebanon. Even with a dire prognosis, she chose to put her life on the line day after day, in the market place, on the streets, and in homes of Moslems, often with the wives of Hezbollah, sharing tea and the love of Jesus.

To others it looks like courage, but to Gale it felt like confidence. Her hope committed her to actions that connected her to God's promises; she knew where she was going and no car bomb or cancer bomb could ever change that. The space vacated by departing worries of this world opened up room for ever more joyful living and always in the present. The future was already secure irrespective of geography, geopolitics or cancer. *"Hope acts on the conviction that God will complete the work He has begun even when the appearances, especially when the appearances, oppose it."*[10]

*Social scientists suggest that most of us who are well spend a third of our time thinking about or worrying about what the future holds—time for the most part wasted. For those with cancer it is even more. Not so for those who believe Jesus' promises and know the future He has for them. Freed from the past and secure in their future, they have 33 percent more time than the worriers to live in the present without actually living one day longer! If you are worried about how long you have to live, why not check out Jesus' promises. Let them settle into your heart and increase your life by 33 percent even before you see any doctor, take any medicine or spend a nickel. The Bible says, "do not be afraid" 127 times and tells you how!*

Gale did. She had stacks of Bible verses (ammunition) around the house which she could frequently be found meditating on. She was one of the Windrunners who was blessed in many ways and outlived her prognosis by years. The biologic certainty that her metastatic malignant melanoma would consume her body never compromised the effervescence of her hopes in this life and beyond.

Gale took all the prescribed treatment including extensive surgery and never abandoned hope that it would work, but it wasn't that hope that sustained her so she could hold it lightly. David marveled: ***"She steadfastly lived with a hope that she'd recover and somehow that hope melded with and was fortified by her hope in Heaven. She was able to look past the boundary of this life to the kingdom we hear, sing and dream about."*** More than once she spoke of how, "the bold line, even the chasm that separates most mortals from the place called heaven seemed to blur more and more each day."

Gale had been like a mom to a university student, who had lived in their home. David overheard her goodbye to Ahmed, "I'm going to Jesus soon..... I want you to come, too." He went on to describe all the tears that flowed: "They were not tears of despair, but on the contrary, tears of great hope—of *anticipation*!"

William Stringfellow's words are again apt and worth repeating ***"Hope is reliance upon grace in the face of death: the issue is that of receiving life as a gift. Not as a reward and not as a punishment; hope is living constantly, patiently, expectantly, resiliently, joyously in the efficacy of the word of God."***[11] Where there is hope, confidence follows and courage comes naturally. With that Eugene Petersen reminds us, "Every person we meet must be drawn into that expectation. If you buy into what you say you believe and have courage, that is your commission."[5]

# DAY 5

# A WINDRUNNER'S JOURNAL

*I invite you to reread every sentence above which is **bold** and in **italics**. Write it down, in your own words if you wish, to remember it, reflect on it, discuss it, or even memorize it.*

_____

_____

_____

_____

_____

_____

_____

_____

_____

_____

_____

_____

_____

_____

# TIME TO WRITE THE REST OF YOUR LIFE'S SCRIPT

Hope is a mysterious thing. Webster defines it as _____
_____.

*What is the biblical definition of hope?*

The only hope I have never seen fail grows out of a close relationship with Jesus. Indeed, it is the very byproduct of that relationship and when you have it you can enjoy holding onto the others, but lightly—no longer desperately. When you are certain of Jesus you can live in peace despite the uncertainties of all the rest.

*Will you take that risk today?*

Another way to practice hope and grow your confidence in God's promises is to get directly and personally involved in His work in your community and in the world.

*Where have you discovered you can become involved in your community and in the world?*

Social scientists suggest that most of us who are well spend a third of our time thinking about or worrying about what the future holds—time for the most part wasted.

*How much time do you spend worrying about the future?*

The Bible says, "do not be afraid" 127 times and tells you how!

*Look these up and use them as part of your arsenal of ammunition against the dragon!*

*Also check out Appendix 1 "Ammunition" for a list of the scriptures that Dave and others have found particularly helpful.*

# CHAPTER 8

# THE HOPE OF HEAVEN - GOD'S ENCORE

**"You never have the ability or courage to stop believing the illusion (holding onto the allure of the world we know) until you have something more and better to take its place."[7]**

## MARY

One evening I found Mary resting on a couch by the fireside and sat by her side. She was recovering from phlebitis in her legs which had sent clots to her lungs; both being complications of the pancreatic cancer that was inexorably withering away her body. Although each hopeful treatment had

---

[7] Richard Rohr and Joseph Martos, *Wild to Wise*, p. 29, Franciscan Media, 2005.

become just another disappointment and the prospects for her Bell Lap were sadly shortening, her spirit never flagged. She held onto the hand of a Lord she knew well ever confident that while His plans for her in this world were winding down He had more for her in the next.

Mary and Al had both known heartbreak before having each endured some of the gritty stuff of life. So when they found each other later in life, it seemed magical and made in Heaven—and I think it was. When her cancer hit with a catastrophic force, it squashed their dreams, doused their joy, and filled their skies with clouds—at first. Then to an observer it became apparent there was something else going on, too; something special, something other worldly, something in and for both of them that I only got to watch from the outside. It was something for which I have no everyday words to describe; perhaps transcendence says it best. I felt it the first time I visited their home and again on that night.

While always lovely, it seemed in that moment that Mary's big blue eyes shown even bigger and her smile even more radiant. Her gaze seemed focused somewhere beyond the ceiling and then she spoke, "I just love thinking about Heaven."

I thought, "Wow, she is not only at peace, but she in reveling in some expectation: God is luring her toward Himself."

Then as if on cue, the strong, but quiet man who is her husband, began singing in a raspy country drawl:

*"This world is not my home*
*I'm just passin' thru*
*If Heaven's not my home*
*Oh Lord, what shall I do?*

*The angels beckon me*
*From Heaven's open door*
*And I can't feel at home*
*In this-here world anymore."*[1]

Married just over a year before with delicious hopes for decades of life together, their separation by a premature death will always seem a tragedy; yet somehow they felt something drawing them through and beyond their tears, something that enriched their lives and their love for one another. It was some kind of hope that heals and strengthens. How can that be?

Wondering how life is for Al two years later, I corralled him for dinner. He told me that the healing hope and strength that grew while at Mary's side still persists. It hasn't changed the fact for him that life is still like a boxing match with round after round of problem encounters, some that you win and others that beat you up, but the blows that land don't wound the way they used to, the strength to go on is heightened and the fear of ever losing the match is gone.

## WHAT'S SO BAD ABOUT DYING?

Bad is not anything Jesus spoke about. *It is the fearful whispers of the Dragon, "You are going to miss out, time is going to run out, what if, not enough, what if...?*

Satan's mighty weapon, the fear of death is about so much more than the actual dying itself. There may be some transient pains or other symptoms during the last days, but *capable* physicians with the aid of a hospice program are able to control them the vast majority of the time—emphasis on *"capable physicians."* Be sure to find one. Expertise varies widely.

However, no bold and capable physician can begin to compete with the wily Dragon's, "Think of all you are going to miss out on," and then he lists countless precious things.

Irrespective of a patients age, many say they just aren't finished with life yet; something is still missing. Even before a life threatening disease interrupts their middle years, many start sensing that something isn't quite right, not what they expected, not what they hoped for. They feel a longing for *something more*: something lost that nostalgia hints at or maybe something they can touch only in their dreams or feel only in the romanticism of movies, music, poetry or a sunset.

There is something intangible we all long for, but can scarcely speak of; so we keep it buried. We feel alone if we dare to think about it seldom recognizing that no one else achieves the completeness they yearn for on their own either no matter how long they live. This side of eternity we all feel lonely, incomplete, searching, and wondering: Is that missing something really on the other side? Is it really worth dying for? Can it compensate for what I am losing? Then along comes cancer and the feelings become more acute—even desperate.

Most of us are clueless about what we may get on the other side in exchange for dying, so how can we possibly know if dying is worth it? Ask the buried seed splitting open in the dark cold earth or the caterpillar entering metamorphosis, or the birth-canal baby whose maternal blood supply is shutting down. Would any of them be excited about a future they cannot see or even imagine? Can an eight-year-old imagine what it is like to be twenty-five, forty, sixty or would they rather leap to the window sill and night sky with Peter Pan. Did we ever want to grow up; for childhood to ever die?

The reality is that we often do not like change, even when it might be for the better. The familiar, no matter how painful, is often preferable because it is known.

Yet "in order to come to a fuller life and spirit we must constantly be letting go of a present life and spirit."[2] Many can testify to that truth. The letting go and moving on may be elective or coerced, but always necessary in order to grab onto something else, and always harder without knowing what next is. The key is looking over the horizon for that new life so as to inspire our reaching expectations.

Most would rather not think about dying let alone talk about it. A study at Stanford University actually demonstrated that most of us don't start thinking about end of life issues until we are within twenty years of reaching it, but Jesus never stopped thinking about it. "He never lost sight of where he was headed—that exhilarating finish in and with God" and why did He keep it in the forefront of His mind? So "he could put up with anything along the way (Hebrews 12:2 MSG).

Life is seldom complete as we chase our ever expanding repertoire of dreams. Every one we catch is soon replaced by another and each desperately held in the bittersweet knowledge that death will amputate them all. However, when our dreams reach out to Heaven, desperation departs replaced by hope and expectancy. Tears flowing and hands wringing shifts to smiles growing and hands reaching for the door into tomorrow.

*The Windrunners defeat the dragon every time with withering irrelevancy by reframing its questions:*

- *What if there is no missing out?*
- *What if God's promises are real?*
- *What if Heaven is everything God says it is?*
- *What if this life is only the hors d'oeuvre that He says it is and the main course and desert are in Heaven with Him as He says it is?*

We know about hors d'oeuvres: they are only meant to pique our appetite, never to satiate or completely satisfy. Still being hungry with a growing appetite is just the way it is meant to be. The Windrunners know that they are not going to miss out on anything and that the fullness of everything and every relationship is yet to come.

Jesus outright tells us, "Don't be afraid of missing out. You are my dearest friends. The Father wants to give you the very Kingdom itself" (Luke 12:32 MSG).

*God doesn't unmake anything. He only completes it; He outright tells us the finest wine to share awaits us. Is there any reason for any more sadness than at the farewell of a daughter boarding a plane for college? There will be a reunion.*

# Day 1

# A Windrunner's Journal

*I invite you to reread every sentence above which is **bold** and in **italics**. Write it down, in your own words if you wish, to remember it, reflect on it, discuss it, or even memorize it.*

_____

_____

_____

_____

_____

_____

_____

_____

_____

_____

_____

_____

_____

## WHAT IS HEAVEN?

*"God usually doesn't replace his original creation, but when he does, He replaces it with something that is far better, never worse."*[3]

> *No eye has seen*
> *No ear has heard*
> *No mind has conceived*
> *What God has prepared for those who love him.*
> (I Corinthians 2:9)

Stories of Heaven are invitations to go there first in your imagination because "while reason is the natural organ of truth, imagination is the organ of meaning." As Heaven by definition is outside our experience, we can only grasp at it by applying our imagination to the symbolism in scripture. That is a worthy undertaking.

**Death is always hard to get acquainted with, so get to know Heaven instead. Then, if you will, by faith, try to see it as your promised home and then you can live in breathless anticipation of your journey's end.** Let knowledge of Heaven beckon you away from the mess of this life and set you on a course toward the next.

All peoples, cultures, and religions throughout time and across the globe have some concept of heaven which shares the presence of a god who is the source of goodness, judgment, and mercy. No leader except Jesus claims to have been there, let alone claims to have created it or to be the author of mercy and judgment. Not surprising, most descriptions apart from the Bible lack detail about the physical nature, purpose, and permanence of Heaven or even the entry criteria, but the Bible tells it all.

Colloquially, people everywhere speak of their postmortem destination as Heaven. In his sermon on heaven, Gino Grunberg said, "How would you like to wake up tomorrow and have the world set right? No more hungry children, no more terrorists, no more broken families or drought, no more violence in the Middle East or racism, no more poverty, illness or death, not just the world made right, but you would be made right. You would speak the truth with courage and love, you would be a great friend, do excellent work, your body would be full of energy and each morning you would be filled with more joy than the morning before."[8] *That is the resurrection power, the resurrected body, and the resurrected life which we can live out in the place called heaven and can look forward to with breathless expectation.*

Some are informed but confused; some consider all religions as just different pathways to the same heavenly destination. However, all religions are not the same: "Muslims believe someone who dies in jihad is martyred and goes straight to Heaven, while the Hindus believe the vigorous outworking of karma requires them to be recycled in a different body to pursue the next stage of their destiny. Buddhists seek to lose their identity in a nameless, formless bliss like an ice cube joining a tropical ocean. Orthodox

---

[8] Gino Grunberg, Sermon on Heaven, 2016

Jews believe in an individual bodily resurrection but only for the righteous."[5] Then there is a somewhat nebulous nature religion (pantheism) which borrows elements of Buddhist thought and relabels it for the New Age. In it one is absorbed into the natural world of sun, wind, earth, and every growing thing. Molecules are simply rearranged into another form, so death never really happens. This creates for them a comforting aura of an everlasting presence in the pulse and beauty of nature.

For those who follow Christ, knowledge of Heaven comes from two sources, God's words through His prophets and God's word made flesh in Jesus. Both were preserved in the early Scriptures and later collated into the Bible and both were endorsed by the historically verified resurrection of Jesus. It is mentioned in fifty-four of the sixty-six books of the Bible.

"Heaven, in the Bible, is not just a future destiny, but the other, hidden dimension of our ordinary life – God's dimension. God made heaven and earth; at the last He will remake both and join them together forever."[6] Today orthodox biblical scholars picture existence in the new Heaven as a vibrant and active human life reflecting God's will and His image in us in new bodies on a new earth, but only for those who have made a genuine commitment to Jesus.

In study of world religions, I don't find any that claim everyone is going to Heaven; there are always entry criteria. "The Universalist point of view is that God is eventually going to work things out so that everyone gets into heaven. (That is not something we're in any position to assure anyone about, however.)"[7]

## FUNDAMENTAL BELL QUESTIONS

*When the bell rings the same fundamental questions confront all of us...*

*What can we expect?*
*What should we fear?*
*What can we hope for?*
*Finally, what should we do?*

We scramble to doctors for answers, or maybe to herbalists, acupuncturist, or quacks. They peddle their wares, science, vitamins, needles, or mystery hogwash to try to deliver on one hope: "Give me back my life on my terms, as I dream of it, unlimited and overflowing."

As one patient put it, "I want my life back...I don't want to die this angry. I don't want this god-awful death that wasn't my fault!"[8] Frightened, they go looking everywhere for some hope to grab onto. They don't insist that the means of their rescue be scientifically proven or valid as long as there is a promise. Curiously, often the promises are enough. Quacks and charlatans know this and exploit it—so do some doctors.

People know that life without hope means only despair; therefore, most will cling fearfully to almost anything, even if it isn't working, rather than give up hoping altogether. The undeniable and extraordinary value of hope is then transferred to whatever the treatment—as if the value of treatment and the value of hope were the same thing. They are not. Yet if another treatment is the only hope offered, then to pass it up could mean having no hope at all.

Hence, when a third or fourth relapse occurs and things are getting desperate, the last treatment option becomes incredibly valuable if it is the only source of hope—even if it is actually medically/biologically worthless. Remember: ***Beware of the physician who doesn't know Jesus or anything about Heaven. He will know only one hope: more treatment. Even if he/she is compassionate, that is all he will have to offer. He will know that no hope is never an option so he will offer it even if it isn't worth much or perhaps worth anything.***

When well, we all can understand this, but when sick and confused, we often dare not think about it. So into that thought-vacuum slithers fear. Just knowing there are a limited number of treatment options and that one day the last one will arrive creates a gaping hole in our security armor giving the dragon and fear direct access to our hearts *well before the last treatment decision is even before us—even while other treatments are still working.* Uninvited, that fearful malaise will arrive, and unchecked, it will fester and grow just as invisible as PTSD and as the hallmark of the living dead.

# DAY 2

# A WINDRUNNER'S JOURNAL

*I invite you to reread every sentence above which is **bold** and in **italics**. Write it down, in your own words if you wish, to remember it, reflect on it, discuss it, or even memorize it.*

_____

_____

_____

_____

_____

_____

_____

_____

_____

_____

_____

_____

_____

## Diversifying Your Portfolio

Is there another way? Might it be good to have a fallback plan when treatment doesn't work, such as a diversified portfolio of hopes? Windrunners do. They would say that having such a plan not only helps them face the end of treatment, but brings a greater peace and vitality to all other treatments even while those are working effectively. Henry, who had been pondering the end of his life, mused, *"If you have got tomorrow figured out (referring to Heaven), it becomes easier to live today."*

It is worth mustering up hopes, goals, and targets for each new day, week, and month. Savor them, and celebrate each one as it is achieved. Add more, yet recognize these are all partial measures destined to be diluted as the hope of ongoing health fades. Thankfully, there is one exception that dwarfs them all and never fades. That is the kaleidoscope of hopes God has for His people in Heaven which is beyond my mind or yours to conceive in its entirety, but entirely possible to conceive in part.

Heaven gets little play on the evening news or Sunday pulpits or in our daily conversations, probably because it congers up the unapproachable death subject. For many of us, it is not until we find ourselves teetering on the precipice between life and death that we dare to look over the edge and consider what is beyond. Hearing the bell ring can change all that. It gets death, the 1000-pound gorilla in the room, right on the table, and with it, consideration of what is to come: Heaven or Hell.

When the busyness of life doesn't leave much room for reflection or study, our concept of reality is limited to our own experience, but it is not—nor is Heaven. So, how can we get excited about something we have never experienced and seldom discussed? Must we travel through the mystery of our lives with only hearsay information or are there clues we are overlooking in our haste? Are there hints the author has woven in the plot, living metaphors hidden right before our eyes waiting for recognition?

Consider the story of a pair of twins in the womb speculating about birth. The first was growing ever eager, the second, ever more anxious, "I like it here. It is warm and safe—it is all I have ever known. Change frightens me." The eager precocious brother responds, "You must be kidding; there is a whole world out there! In here it's all dark, out there, there is light and something they call Technicolor. In here all we can hear is the lub dub, lub dub of Mom's heart. Outside there are orchestras and rock bands. There are mountains and oceans and other people like us only bigger. There we can run and jump, ski and surf, play baseball and football, and dance to the music. Here you can't roll over without kicking me. As soon as we leave here, we get to join the big people in that world and even meet our mother." The anxious twin just scrunched up his face and retorted, ***"You are crazy bro. Get real. I doubt there is a mother and I'm sure there's no life after birth!"***[9]

Before one endures every unnecessary possible side effect of medical treatment, every fearful failure or goes running blindly into the arms of one false hope or another, one had best know about the alternative hope that never fails, Heaven. After all, how can the *hopes of Heaven* lift one above the concerns of earth if one doesn't know anything about them? How can one be motivated for a journey if the directions and the destination are unknown? That is why I wrote this chapter. Jesus is the road. Heaven is the destination.

## STORY WITHIN A STORY

A whole life is as an hour in the story of eternity and sometimes an hour within a day can hold the whole story of life: Kids play building sand castles at the beach, ever adding more detail, a turret, a causeway, a moat, their imaginations reeling ever ahead of their construction. Amused parents look on. The tide turns inward and waves creep ever closer. Little actions become more frenetic building protective walls and dams. Tensions rise. Tired kids begin to squabble. Vigilant parents offer advice and consolation hoping the kids will figure it out and take steps towards growing up. A hit here, a swat there, sand to the back, sand to the face. Waves erode castle walls, whining crescendos, tears flow, only one solution for a savvy parent: swoop in at the right moment and whisk them away to a safe home, a warm bath, fresh clothes, hot chocolate, and a nap. Is the author of our stories trying to tell us something through our lives?

It has been said we have two lives: "The life we learn with and the life we live with after that."[10] Use yours. Messages are there waiting to be discovered.

Have you ever noticed how fast a distraught child, if distracted, can go from tears to laughter? The entire trauma that begot the tears is forgotten, erased by something new when it is delivered with love and security. Hopefully, in the course of it all they learned something. I wonder if God is any less amused with us and our sandbox-lives. He assures us of our Heavenly home and rewards: the new clothes, the nap, and chocolate, but do we believe Him? Will we know Him and trust Him when He comes to pick us up? (Chapter 2)

Hints are all around us in the metaphors of our lives. Remember the wonderful childhood expectations of Christmas and Santa Claus? We didn't understand it all at first, but we knew it was special and our hopes were electrifying; so high that we would give up playing to go to bed early hoping to bring morning and Santa sooner. Parents would help build the excitement. Is there a parallel here? God's Word tells us, "The created world itself can hardly wait for what's coming next. Everything in creation is being more or less held back. God reins it in until creation and all the creatures are ready and can be released into the glorious times ahead. Meanwhile, the joyful anticipation deepens" (Romans 18-21 MSG).

Notice in yourself how the power of anticipation is lost as soon as you hear the word "maybe." God knows this so His words in Scripture are unequivocal on this point, check them out (see

Appendix 111—*What Does Scripture Say About Heaven)*. If you are to enjoy living in the expectancy of Heaven, you need to be confident Heaven is real and it is where you are bound. Joyful anticipation is infectious; surround yourself with others who have it and be sure to pass it on. It is what the homestretch is about.

Most of us can attest to the motivational power of a reward in proportion to its size and proximity. It can be real or imagined, positive or negative. The motivation is kindled by a spark of desire or dread and fanned by God with hope or by Satan with lust or fear.

**Satan may think God's hopes are silly and no match for his powers of fear and deceit. He is absolutely correct for those who do not know Jesus and His promises** that apply to this life and the next. However, those who know, "rejoice in that day and leap for joy, because great is the reward in heaven" (Luke 6:23).

## APPROACHING WHAT SCRIPTURE SAYS, BUT HOW

Scriptural truth is timeless and universal. It speaks to us individually and collectively, both in the first century and in the twenty-first. What we have learned in 2000 years may add to the depth of our understanding, but it cannot negate how it would have been understood in the first century. Hence, when we come to the Bible to learn about Heaven and Hell, we bring the thesaurus of our own experience with God alongside the historical perspective of God's experience with the Hebrews. We use both to come up with an interpretation of scripture which is sometimes literal, sometimes figurative and hopefully, all together divine.

No one but a mathematician speaks with an expectation that they will be understood absolutely literally, and no one but the artist speaks with the expectation that they will be taken absolutely figuratively. The poet and the punster rely on the intrigue between the two and so does God.

We speak figuratively when words alone are insufficient to carry the requisite subtlety or complexity of our subject and then we rely on the prior knowledge and the creative ingenuity of the listener. We require active participation of the listener to engage their imagination to grasp much of what we are saying. That is exactly what Jesus and the prophets expected of their listeners and of us as we read their words. Spanish Bible scholar Luis Alonso Schokel reminds us, "What has been written with imagination must be interpreted with imagination."[16] Recognizing God is doing the best He can within the limits of our abilities, we need not limit Him further by not using them.

We are wrong if we elect to reside trapped within our own limited perceptions of time and space and arrogantly dare to understand scripture only in our own finite terms. Even in a single lifetime space has contracted and time has expanded: the moon is now within man's reach and he can cross a continent between breakfast and dinner. Both achievements were beyond the finite imagination a lifetime ago.

God exists outside time and space and He invites us to step out to Him - at least with our imaginations. "Heaven is by definition outside our experience, but all intelligible descriptions must be of things within our experience."[12]

*There is no vocabulary to describe what heaven holds, but instead of leaving us with a void, God gives us clues and metaphors and sometimes events in history. Then He gives us imagination to weave them all together into a divine hologram rather like projecting God's 5-D love picture of Himself and Heaven onto the 4-D surface of our minds.*

"Now we see things imperfectly as in a clouded mirror, but then we will see everything with perfect clarity" (or in Greek: see face to face) (1 Corinthians 13:12 MSG). "No eye has seen, no ear has heard, and no mind has imagined what God has prepared for those who love him" (1 Corinthians 2:9.) While we can scarcely conceive His promises, He never says don't try to imagine them. Indeed, He sparks our imaginations with His clues.

He knows we will bite. Is there anything more compelling than a secret closely held coupled with a promise of revelation in the future? That is exactly what God has done with His creation. To those who are listening, everything around us whispers, "There is more, there is **more**, there **IS** more." Then the ingenious, the explorers, and the scientists discover more. Still the whisper continues and draws every listener with an imagination onward. It could seem teasingly wicked, but to those who listen, God promises to tell all (Matthew 10:39 and see Appendix III:35).

# DAY 3

# A WINDRUNNER'S JOURNAL

*I invite you to reread every sentence above which is **bold** and in **italics**. Write it down, in your own words if you wish, to remember it, reflect on it, discuss it, or even memorize it.*

_____

_____

_____

_____

_____

_____

_____

_____

_____

_____

_____

_____

_____

# WHY DOES HE WAIT?

Perhaps it is to give us time to train our ears, eyes, and minds to better hear, see, and imagine. The novice first exposed to orchestral music or fine art, or who sips a cellared Bordeaux wine or an aged whiskey is seldom able to appreciate the full richness of the experience. With every return visit they become able to taste more, hear more, the overlapping melodies, changes in rhythm, timber, and cadence. You taste the hint of black cherry, pepper or oak, or the peat of the Isle of Islay and the salt air off Dundee. I just wonder whether God is giving those who pay attention time to develop their pallet so that the rewards of heaven will be that much greater—and "to let the anticipation grow."

As kids, we knew the sharing of a deep secret was not a casual or reckless affair, but a brokered contract of fidelity, sealed by an oath "on your mother's grave" or mixed blood from knife pricked thumbs or some such vow. Child's play? Not really. God does the same. He says, "Give Me your heart and I will tell you. I'll even show you all My secrets some now and some later."

The some now is an experience of His Kingdom life and the peace that goes with it. The some later is every mystery of His creation and Himself and His Heaven. If you haven't given Him your whole heart, these are only words with little meaning, like the words "ice cream" to the aborigine—unimaginable and meaningless. Wendell knew the "some now" and I'm sure he is being enchanted every day in Heaven with "all later," unending revelations—never a dull moment.

I am not saying Heaven is a creation of our collective imagination, although as a child I wasn't so sure. Throughout my youth, I heard references to Heaven but they seemed on par with Santa Claus, the Easter Bunny, and the Tooth Fairy; pretty much something out of storybooks and Grimm's Fairy Tales. My parents were serious about it, but they were also serious about, "you better not pout, you better not cry, you better not shout, I'm telling you why: Santa Claus is coming to town." It was mostly about fun, with a little benign parental manipulation thrown in. Elves were watching before Christmas regarding my worthiness for presents and I supposed the Angels were keeping their scorecards the rest of the time with an entrance into heaven in the balance.

***However, I have come to learn that Heaven is real and that it's not about performance and reward. It's about a promise with a purpose.***

So what does this promise look like, feel like, and play out like?

## THE PROMISE OF HEAVEN: WHAT DOES SCRIPTURE TELL US?

Finding a description for love in the Bible is easy compared to finding one of Heaven and Hell. There is no concise, comprehensive chapter on Heaven or Hell. Descriptions are scattered all over the Old and New Testaments. I've often wondered why the difference.

I'm left with two conclusions. The first is that it is essential to understand love as early in life as possible so it is spoon fed to us in I Cor 13. Whereas knowledge of Heaven is not needed until much later, and being a more complex subject needs a more seasoned mind to understand it. Perhaps such knowledge is both a privilege and a blessing. Perhaps it is meant to be pursued so that it is with the pursuit that one is blessed and with the blessing comes hope, and with hope comes the endurance for the far corner and a home stretch of the Bell Lap. Remember Hebrews 12:2 where **Jesus *"never lost sight of where he was headed"*** so "He could put up with *anything* along the way: the cross, shame, *whatever*." We, too, need to never lose sight of where we are headed so we can endure and hold fast to the One who calls us.

The quintessential feature of Heaven is the presence of Jesus (APPENDIX III:6), and our unfettered relationship with Him through which we finally find a freedom from the bondage of our wounds, peace, security, understanding, excitement, feasting, and joy (APPENDIX III: 21). We will live there both in space and time and have meaningful life, relationships, positions, and purpose (APPENDIX III: 15, 13, 18). Heaven is a physical place (APPENDIX III: 1, 2, 7, 11, 40), where we will not just exist suspended in eternity as spirit vapors in the clouds, nor as inanimate rocks on the ground, nor as androgynous automatons. We will have new, unique, transformed physical bodies (APPENDIX

III: 25) on a material new Earth (APPENDIX III: 1, 2), both similar, and both better than the bodies and earth we know today. He has given us Yosemite in the spring, the Tetons in the fall, Yellowstone in winter, the Grand Canyon, the Karakoram, the Serengeti, along with Bach, the Beatles, and the female mystique all just to wet our appetite for what lies ahead in Heaven for us to discover and enjoy.

Every good thing in this life which brings us meaning, adventure, intrigue, and fulfillment will be present, but better. To me that means the powder snow for skiing will be deep and dry, the mountains for climbing rugged and steep, the chocolate dark and rich, the trout large and wily, the firesides cozy, the port tawny, the scotch peaty, the quiche savory, the apples juicy, the melodies ethereal, and the vista's magnificent. Because there is not a word for the superlatives that await us, we are given hints to feed our imaginations.

Scripture doesn't mention skiing, scotch or chocolate, but Jesus did say to His disciples, "I confer on you the royal authority my father conferred on me so you can eat and drink at my table and be strengthened" (Luke 22: 30). Isaiah 25:6 says, "On this mountain the Lord Almighty will prepare a feast of rich food for all peoples, a banquet of aged wine – the best meats and the finest wines," and we know that when Jesus turned water to wine at the wedding feast in Cana it wasn't Thunderbird. It was what the sommelier called the "finest." As God has made it all, from the snow to grapes, it seems reasonable to imagine it all will be superb.

*C.S. Lewis, Oxford professor, Christian apologist, theologian, and academic, holding tight to scripture tells us there are four things we can expect when we get to Heaven: "The symbols under which Heaven is presented us are a wedding, a city, a concert, and a dinner party."*

**A wedding, beautiful and perfect:** Revelation 19:6-7 says, "The wedding of the lamb has come and his bride has made herself ready." The bride is us.

**A city:** Revelation 21:1-5 says, "The new Jerusalem.... God's dwelling place among the people and he will dwell with them.... He will wipe away every tear from their eyes. There will be no more death or morning or crying or pain." It is a place in which we are living, creating, celebrating, and worshipping.

**A dinner party:** Matthew 22:1 says, "The kingdom of heaven is like a king who prepared a wedding banquet for his son..." an epic party you don't want to miss. Family dinners are a slice of heaven, the love and laughter, engaging ideas, honoring one another, good food and wine. Heaven will be even more with our deepest needs fulfilled. The King has been sending out invitations for 2000 years to join in the resurrected body of Jesus in a place named Heaven, the wedding, the concert, and the dinner party. Say, "Yes!"

One thing that isn't there is competition of the sort that demeans a looser or elevates a winner. We all die powerless— with a kind of ultimate poverty— a momentary union with all humanity — all those who have died and will die, a communion with all of God's people in Heaven where power and riches are irrelevant, where society is no longer stratified by prowess or beauty, where bigger/better, more/less have no meaning. What a comforting thought to no longer need to compete to get ahead or to watch your back to avoid being overtaken or taken out. Where real and genuine, true and safe have no opposite!

One of my patients lamented, "Don't you imagine Heaven will be boring?" I have heard that question often. It has got to be the most common and disconcerting thought of all who are adventuresome, fun-loving, creative, intellectual, and imaginative— which is most of us. The answer is that there is no hint of that in Scripture. "This resurrection life you received from God is not a timid, grave tending life. It's adventurously expectant, greeting God with a childlike 'What's next Papa?'" (Romans 8:15).

That goes for every good area of endeavor, intellectual, relational, artistic, and physical. He put those passions within us, as well as the estrogen and testosterone. He does not unmake us for Heaven, rather He enables us to fully experience who He created us to be. To borrow John Eldrege's line, "Adventure, with all its requisite danger and wildness is a deeply spiritual longing written in the soul of man." God is not going to take that away just when He gives you a new body and a new earth. Adventure, sport, recreation, games are all God's creations and most are intensely relational. I expect to find them all in Heaven.

When God gives us new bodies, they will still be unique, but healed and whole. However, there is no suggestion we will all be superheroes able to make music like Mozart, paint like Picasso or jump like Jordan. The diversity of our anatomy should facilitate competition while the harmony of our hearts and the satisfied equality of our egos must eliminate pride and shame from the equation of winning and losing. Won't it all be fascinating to discover!

Then my friend asked, "What is adventure without risk? Isn't it risk that energizes adventure? Wouldn't adventure be boring without it?" Risk taking is not inherently sinful and it does seem that God has created many men and some women hardwired for it. Likewise, achievement is a motive that energizes risk taking, but so are prideful proving themselves, getting ahead, and showing off. Perhaps we will be so comfortably sufficient in our identities and status that risk-taking will not be needed. Whatever the reason, Heaven must exist and be wonderful without it, because scripture tells us that risk's downside consequence: pain, is gone, and the upside, achievement is unnecessary. *Perhaps it is that the sufficiency of God trumps our insufficiency and our human concepts of insufficiency (not enough) simply evaporates or are left behind in the grave.*

Jesus spoke, "Do not let your heart be troubled. Trust in God; trust in me. In my father's house are many rooms; if it were not so I would've told you. I am going there to prepare a place for you. And if I go and prepare a place for you, I will come back and take you to be with me that you also may be where I am. You know the way to the place where I am going" (John 14:1–24).

# Day 4

# A Windrunner's Journal

*I invite you to reread every sentence above which is **bold** and in **italics**. Write it down, in your own words if you wish, to remember it, reflect on it, discuss it, or even memorize it.*

_____

_____

_____

_____

_____

_____

_____

_____

_____

_____

_____

_____

## BEYOND IMAGERY

**The promises of heaven may be reduced to just one: we shall be with Christ.** Because Jesus is more than a person and lest our imaginations be limited by our own meager experiences of personhood, true love, and relational ecstasy, we are given a kaleidoscope of earthly imagery to entrance us with our promised future home.

Don't let your ponderings on the amazing blessings of Heaven, health, and the new life take your attention off of Christ, the author and essence of it all. The prizes of Heaven are only windows into the character of our triune God.

We dare not let all visual and experiential imagery distract us from the gracious divinity of Christ; that must be our central image. That is entirely dependent upon the substance of the relationship we have had with Jesus. For those who little know Him, the thought of His company can at best be intellectually speculative based upon the testimonies of friends and Scripture; at worst it could be frightening. Only for those who have intimately engaged Jesus, listened to His voice, risked following His promptings and experienced His divinity can there be excitement to experience more of Him.

I don't find descriptions of working in salt mines or scrubbing floors or a litany of meaningless chores described anywhere in Scripture about Heaven. Instead we find descriptions of rejoicing, feasting, celebrating— food, song, dance, relationships, and purposeful work— prayer, worship, and ongoing discovery. Noting this, Rob Bell points out that in the gospel records of Jesus' life what He does almost as much as teaching and healing was eating long meals. Rob continues, "As Christians, it is our duty to master the art of the long meal" as it is good preparation for Heaven. That is something we can all work on together.

There is also "an enormous wealth of imagery (about our life in Heaven) that we shall have 'glory' which seems to suggest fame, but not fame conferred by our fellow creatures – fame with God, approval or (I might say) 'appreciation' by God."[12] After concluding that, C. S. Lewis goes on to remind us that no one enters Heaven except as a child and that there is nothing so obvious in a child as its great and undisguised pleasure when being praised by its father. Imagine "to be an ingredient in the divine happiness... to be delighted in as an artist delights in his work or a father in a son." Oh, that we might one day hear, "Well done, thou good and faithful servant." However, ere you crumple in feelings of inadequacy, remember we all come as children and I, for one have yet to meet a perfect child, yet all are afforded lots of parental grace, another living metaphor of what the children of God can expect.

**Who Is Invited?** Everyone

**Who Actually Gets In?** *Entry Criteria*

Dallas Willard points out, "Of course, it is not God's will that anyone perish, God is not trying to keep people out of heaven. He is trying to get them into heaven. Some people think that God is sort of up there with His foot against the door, unwilling to let people in. Well, He is willing, but the issue is can you stand to be there? And if you made it, would it be heaven to you, or would it be something much worse?"[17] Would you really want to be constantly in the presence of the God and godly people you may have been rejecting all your life?

Those who accept Jesus' invitation are in and want to be there: "I am the way, and the truth, and the life No one comes to the Father except through me (John 14:6). *If you confess with your mouth that Jesus is Lord and believe in your heart that God raised Him from the dead, you will be saved* (Romans 10:9). "Not everyone who says to me, 'Lord, Lord,' will enter the kingdom of heaven, but the one who does the will of my Father who is in heaven" (Matthew 7:21).

The apostle Thomas just didn't get it. He had no idea where Jesus was going (Heaven) and queried how to get there. "Jesus answered; I am the way" (John 14:5-6) or in essence "follow Me and everything about Me." Later Jesus very specifically describes to whom He will show "the way." It is to those who love Him. Then He tells us, "Whoever has my commands and obeys them, he is the one who loves me." Then He goes one better and tells us that we are not going to have to go hunting around for this place and risk getting lost. He's going to bring it to us! "If anyone loves me he will obey my teaching. My father will love him, and we will come to him and make our home with him." This house with many rooms is coming to those who love Him. Now let that stir your imagination!

The only universal entry criterion is death, but more than just death of the body. For the Christian, Scripture would seem to suggest that death is a two-stage process, one psychologic, the other physiologic. New life comes after the first stage while still in a mortal body and with it comes a reassurance that the second will be no more than stepping through the looking glass (I Corinthians 13:12). The first dying is to oneself, surrendering control of our agendas in life in order to take on the likeness and purposes of Christ. The second is only the surrendering of a worn-out body in this world in exchange for a new body in the next. The whole process starts with one decision, and then plays out over a lifetime culminating with a graduation/commencement exercise: physical death, when an immortal soul only blinks and physical life begins anew in God's dimension.

In 1633, John Donne put it poetically this way: "Death, be not proud, though some have called thee mighty and dreadful, for thou art not so. For those whom thou thinkest thou dost overthrow die not, poor Death, nor yet canst thou kill me... One short sleep past, we wake eternally, and death shall be no more. Death, thou shalt die."[15]

The central New Testament truth is that although death is an enemy, it has been defeated. Those committed to Jesus will be resurrected in new bodies. Commitment to Jesus is not as easy as it sounds. It takes repeatedly asking for Jesus' input on decision making and then the patience to wait for it, the astuteness to perceive it and the will to follow it (Chapter 2). Then you can spit in the eye of death. Windrunners do.

*Death will not win. It does not get to destroy our bodily existence and leave only our souls floating in an ether —like heaven. It does continue to rule in this life for those who cannot or will not take the first step of dying to self. They will continue to struggle to hold on to control of their stiff-necked, self-centered agendas. The cost of obstinacy is an ever-present fear of that unpredictable day when death will take it all away. Deep down, though oft denied, they know there is nothing they can do to prevent it. Deep down they are already resigned to defeat! Finishing weak!*

## THE KINGDOM OF GOD

The kingdom of God is like a king who throws a wedding feast for his son, but it is God who is throwing the feast. It is ready now and we are all invited. As soon as we start making excuses for not accepting the invitation it means we believe we *deserve* to go, but that is where we are mistaken. It is only His grace and great affection that gets us the invitation and it is only an egocentric darkness that prevents us from accepting it.

It's not just a destination on the other side of death, but an eternal Kingdom can start now in **this life** the moment God's character and promises are fully apprehended. It is life full of passion and purpose, adventure and discovery, loving and fearless, full of humor and laughter, worry free, grateful, and secure. Heaven is not a reward kingdom for the well behaved, but an expansion of God's kingdom on earth for those who love Him. And what makes it possible is the loving planning and presence of Jesus. It is only that reveling unconditional love that was and is the essential character of the triune God: Father, Son, and Holy Spirit that existed before we were created and into which we are invited.

Is not our whole life experience in search of that love? Is not everything we do an effort to acquire it? If we lived without anyone to relate to, would we care about the shape of our bodies, the style of our clothes, our cars, homes, jewelry, bank accounts, and even how athletic, skilled, sexy, or smart we are? What if, instead, it was about expressing and receiving love without having to earn or finagle it?

*When you figure out that all you have been searching for is exactly what awaits you in Heaven, the dragon loses his fire and his claws. He becomes powerless and irrelevant. Death is only the door into a love fest with the very source of all love and with every other person who was, is, and will be drawn to it. Now that is something to hold onto with breathless expectation!*

## EXPERIENCING ASSURANCE

It's not about earning a place, passing a test, knowing all about Jesus or signing up. Doug was dying feeling helpless and alone. He had grown up in the church, knew the liturgy and the scriptural basis for hope in the Lord, and he could recite powerful prayers learned in his youth. However, all this knowledge was not enough. God seemed far off, impersonal, and out of reach. Doug's spiritual mechanics were spot on, but none of the prayers he had learned fit his circumstances and he had never just fallen to his knees to bare his heart. He was ripe for a spiritual pilgrimage and a real encounter with Jesus. I wish he could have met Juanita for whom prayer was the lifeblood of her victorious confrontation with cancer and the dragon.

Heaven is the seventh word in the Bible, "In the beginning God created the heavens and the earth" (Genesis 1:1). It is mentioned in 54 of the 66 books in the Bible, seventy times in Matthew alone. For more about the character of heaven and what to expect there, see Appendix III - *What Will Heaven Be Like?* and Appendix IV – *What Does Scripture Say About Heaven?*

# A Windrunner's Journal

*I invite you to reread every sentence above which is **bold** and in **italics**. Write it down, in your own words if you wish, to remember it, reflect on it, discuss it, or even memorize it.*

_____

_____

_____

_____

_____

_____

_____

_____

_____

_____

_____

_____

_____

_____

# TIME TO WRITE THE REST OF YOUR LIFE'S SCRIPT

When our dreams reach out to Heaven, desperation departs replaced by hope and expectancy. Jesus outright tells us, "Don't be afraid of missing out. You are my dearest friends. The Father wants to give you the very Kingdom itself" (Luke 12:32 MSG).

For those who follow Christ, knowledge of Heaven comes from two sources, God's words through His prophets and God's word made flesh in Jesus. Both were preserved in the early Scriptures and later collated into the Bible and both endorsed by the historically verified resurrection of Jesus. It is mentioned in fifty-four of the sixty-six books of the Bible.

See Appendix III: *What Does Scripture Say About Heaven?*

Write out the verses that mean the most to you:

*What are the hints God has woven into the Bible to help us better understand heaven?*

Jesus is the road. Heaven is the destination. It's not about earning a place, passing a test, knowing all about Jesus or signing up.

*So what is it about?*

# CHAPTER 9

# THE ROADWORK – PRAYER

Training for runners involves a lot of roadwork and for Windrunners that equals prayer. It is the very lifeblood of a relationship with Jesus and the universal habit of those who are outrunning the illness that cancer breeds. God knows answers that come before there are questions often fall on deaf ears, so He is always waiting to respond whenever we can formulate a question.

For me, prayer begins with the recognition that He is God and I am not. He is all sufficient and I am not. I need help and He wants to give it. Over and over He invites us to call out to Him when we are out of answers and out of luck, at our wits end or the end our rope. He promises He will either calm the storm or take us through it. He also invites us to talk with Him about every little thing, the minutia and the trivia. We helped our kids put their socks on as well as bandaging their wounds. They are all opportunities for relationship. Sure He may laugh, but He will also answer.

Prayer is a conversation that goes directly to the source: the person and spirit of Jesus who, for the Windrunners, has come to captivate their hearts and minds, and to inhabit their every breath and thought. This chapter will focus on the human side of the conversation and the next one on what we can expect from a God who wants to enter into the healing process. If you are early in your prayer experience, then this is exactly where you want to be, whereas if you are seasoned in prayer you might best skip to the next chapter but skim this one as there may still be a few pearls as it relates to cancer.

When as a layman I speak about prayer it seems most useful to start exactly where I am, not so much presuming to instruct as to compare notes from the trenches of cancer warfare and my own life. I have shared fearsome foxholes with desperate people who are just learning to pray and with some mighty prayer warriors seasoned by past conflicts. If any of our stuff is like your stuff, perhaps these experiences will speak to you.

There is only one unimpeachable authority on how to talk to God and that is the only one to claim He is God's Son and then went on to prove it, Jesus. So quoting Him, then His disciples and the prophets seems a good place to start. Then I will share discoveries from those living through the raw and real everyday stuff of life. These discoveries speak to what you can expect of prayer and when, how, and why.

## JESUS PRAYED

> *"When you pray, do not be like the hypocrites, for they love to pray standing in the synagogues and on the street corners to be seen by men... When you pray, go into your room, close the door and pray to your Father who is unseen. Then when your Father who sees what is done in secret will reward you. And when you pray, do not keep on babbling like pagans, for they think they will be heard because of their many words. Do not be like them, for your Father knows what you need before you ask him. This, then, is how you should pray: 'our father in heaven, hallowed be your name, your kingdom come, your will be done on earth as it is in heaven. Give us today our daily bread. Forgive us our debts, as we have forgiven our debtors. And lead us not into temptation, but deliver us from the evil one.' For if you forgive men when they sin against you, your heavenly father will also forgive you. But if you do not forgive men their sins, your father will not forgive your sins."* (Matthew 6:5)

Note the Lord's Prayer is both a specific prayer and an instructive model emphasizing intimacy, thankfulness, and forgiveness, but also petitioning imperatives: "Give us, forgive us, lead us, and deliver us." It recruits divine participation in our human struggle with evil and temptation and is a wonderful place to start, but then move on in your own words from the heart of your situation both boldly and patiently.

Jesus also prayed, "If you believe, you will receive whatever you ask for in prayer" (Matthew 21:22). Then in Gethsemane before His crucifixion, Jesus prayed, "Abba, Father, everything is possible for you. Take this cup from me. Yet, not what I will, but what you will" (Mark 14:36).

There is a tension in modeling Jesus' self-will-relinquishing words, "thy kingdom come, thy will be done," as well as His Gethsemane prayer, "not what I will, but what you will," and in Matthew 18:19, 21:22, and Mark 11:23 which encourages us to expect miraculous responses, "to anything you ask" or "whatever you ask with faith." In that lies a mystery that compels both to be considered together.

**Paul prayed,** "Be joyful in hope, patient in affliction, faithful in prayer" (Romans 12:12). "Do not be anxious about anything, but in everything, by prayer and petition, with thanksgiving present your request to God and the peace of God, which transcends all understanding, will guard your hearts and your minds in Christ Jesus" (Philippians 4:6).

**James prayed,** "The prayer offered in faith will make the sick person well; the Lord will raise him up... The prayer of a righteous man is powerful and effective" (James 5:15).

**Moses prayed,** "The Lord our God is near to us whenever we pray to him" (Deuteronomy 4:7).

**Other early biblical authors prayed,** "If my people...will humble themselves and pray and seek my face and turn from their wicked ways, then I will hear from heaven and will forgive their sin and heal their land" (2 Chronicles 7:14). "Let everyone who is godly pray" (Psalms 32:16). "The Lord the tests the sacrifice of the wicked, but the prayer of the upright pleases him" (Proverbs 15:8). "The Lord is far from the wicked but he hears the prayers of the righteous" (Proverbs 15:29).

## FOOTBALL AND THE BIBLE

Knowing the Bible is like knowing the playbook and rules of the game before going out on the field, but if you want to actually play football you need to first huddle-up and hear what play is being called. Prayer is the huddle up, the petition for instruction for a play adapted for the particular circumstances on the field, in your life right now.

This is not a bad metaphor in the sense that despite our petitions for God to act, He seldom, whiz-bang, does it all on His own, although He could. He wants us to get involved and to play a specific role so He can move the ball, the issue of our concern and His kingdom, down the field. If we don't listen-up in the huddle, we're unlikely to play our role on the field and the ball won't move forward, nor will His kingdom.

**When?** "Be joyful always, pray **continuously**, give thanks in all circumstances, for this is God's will for you in Christ Jesus" (1 Thessalonians 5:16-18, emphasis added). In the early stages of prayer life, most find their prayers to be self-centered and only in times of need (foxhole Christians like me). With time they become other-focused, yet still only in moments of need. Somewhere I stumbled on a new idea (new to me) described above in 1 Thessalonians 5 where we are encouraged in no uncertain terms to pray continuously.

I could not quite grasp that though I had tried. I'd tried praying over every decision on every patient, every interpretation on every lab value, and on every x-ray finding while walking the hospital halls and everywhere I went. It was exhausting and I seldom sensed a reply fast enough for my needs. Before long I got distracted and returned expeditiously to problem solving on my own. Eventually, I gave up concluding that continuous prayer *didn't work* for me. There just wasn't enough time, or that there was something I was missing, or I just didn't get it, or all three.

I'm not sure what "it *working*" would look like. I think I expected immediate results. I'd had a number of extraordinary immediate answers to prayers in the consultation room with patients sitting in front of me. They were usually at the end of their rope and so was I. They usually had failed every treatment

I could imagine or had come up with a new symptom that thoroughly confused me. Clueless and helpless, I would keep asking them questions while frantically praying silently. Then, out of the blue, an amazing new idea or solution would pop in my head. God had clearly showed up and fast. So, with continuous prayer I expected God to show up fast every time and to become a micromanager giving me feedback on every diddle and daddle or at least an "atta-boy" or a "right on" when I was on the correct track or "whoa— try again soldier" if I wasn't. Better yet I expected an out right answer, but none of that happened.

Sometimes just formulating the question in prayer focuses my attention keenly enough that I realize I already know part of the answer. **Part of God's intention has been to bring clarity to the question.**

## WHY PRAY?

In the next stage of my prayer adventure, I concluded that prayer isn't just about results I could see or hear. It was simply one component of my relationship with God. Some of it is just about information transfer and sharing life, a lot like another mysterious relationship in my life— the one with my wife. The fabric of our relationship consists of many threads— some get responses, some don't. The words are important, but facial expressions, touch, body language, and something out in cyberspace called intuition, are every bit as important. These go beyond words to convey my thoughts to her and hers to me using all our senses; they go deeper.

I would hardly expect a response to every intentional or incidental message I sent to her, yet they are all part of our relationship, so I concluded it must be the same with God. Perhaps, He is already watching and He already knows what is going on in my head and heart just like I do when I see a certain smile on my wife's face. However, I still appreciate when she reaches out for me.

I believe God is like that. He loves us to reach for Him in prayer. **He already knows our need, but when we pray it tells Him we recognize it and are ready to listen.** More importantly it compels us to define our need and prepares our minds to pay attention and our souls to listen.

I concluded that God no more intends to respond immediately or verbally to my every prayer than my wife does to my every expression or gesture; He receives them all, but sometimes His response is not to respond yet.

Then I came to believe that for me "continuous" means continuous grateful conversation recognizing His blessings and provisions in my life coupled with continuous active submission to His will as best I can figure it out. I concluded (albeit incorrectly) that I was pretty much on my own a lot of the time and wasn't going to hear from Him much and it would be pretty clear when I did.

This is a pretty easy place for a guy to go. Many of us do not value, understand or trust nonverbal communication. The "guess what I am thinking approach" that some of the female gender (not my wife) have been known to perfect often doesn't work with us. Whereas the: "tell it like it is, use words, something I can hear and understand" approach really does. I must have figured God to be pretty much a guy (at least in pictures and pronouns) so that is what I expected.

Well, I was wrong on this one, too. That stance is as off-base and ineffective with God as it is with ladies. The more I get to know the women in my life, the more I suspect that one of the reasons God created them as He did, and blessed us with them as He does, is to show us something about Himself. The prayer arena would seem to be one of many where the analogy applies.

He wants us to listen actively not just with our ears, but with our hearts, souls, intuitions, and everything that is within us. In my experience, He speaks a whole lot more often than I ever imagined, but it is with whispers, nudges, cajoling, wooing, events, and even other people or an occasional bear. If He has suggestions, they are often soft. If He is exasperated, it seems His voice is much louder and often in the form of unfortunate, albeit instructive, natural consequences He foresees and does not prevent.

So, where I try to be now starts with continuous grateful recognition of His blessings and provisions, continuous submission followed by continuous active listening. I find the enemy attacks me on all fronts. He tries to overshadow the blessings by creating ever-expanding new needs and desires. He highlights disappointments to be sure I shamefully remember them and he tries to defeat my commitment to submit by drumming up feelings of "I deserve" and "it's not fair." To prevent my listening, he throws in the urgencies of business, patient care, and my own agendas. If he succeeds, I become discontent, bitter, and out of time for my agenda and out of time for prayer or listening and therefore clueless about his agenda. Enemy wins.

Continuous prayer means keeping Him in the forefront of our minds and in the midst of our relationships. It means recruiting others to pray for us and then listening to what they hear. Including them in our dialog with God increases the power of our prayers, enriches our friendships, and increases the number of antennae on alert to receive what God is trying to say. In community His voice can become clearer.[1]

Of course, all that is heard also needs to be sifted through God's Word in the scriptures. Although He does not speak directly to every imaginable issue, He reveals His character and attitudes consistently; they don't change. If what we think we hear is not in harmony with His voice in scripture, we had better listen some more.[1]

## FOR PROTECTION AND BLESSING

**"God's love is unconditional, but His favor and blessings are not."[2] Neither is His protection**. Scripture is clear that we are responsible to make certain decisions and to be in communication with Him to receive all He promises. Grace (undeserved favor) is His independent prerogative, but becoming eligible for His promises is our responsibility. Salvation depends on our decision. Blessings and protection depend at least in part upon our communication.

We need not split hairs on this. He does bless and protect those He loves without our asking. Hallelujah! However, the closer we are in contact with Him, the more that is possible. It helps me to recall going out in the woods with my dad as a small boy. His love for me and his willingness to guide and protect me were huge and obvious. If I wandered off on my own, out of earshot, without communicating with him, I left my dad in no position to direct or safeguard me. It's not a perfect metaphor for my relationship with God, but it's close.

God gives us total free will, more than most fathers give their kids. When we behave like two-year-olds, "I do it myself," He lets us until we ask/pray for His oversight or intervention. It is our responsibility to stay close. **The best tactic is to tell Him where you're going and what you hope to achieve, and to ask Him to go along. Better yet, ask Him if it is a good idea and which way to head out.** It means a lot to Him, just as it does to us when our children ask us for advice or to come along. God is always a gentleman and gentlemen don't go where they are not invited.

Sometimes I spend time with high school kids in Young Life out in the barn to talk about life and God. One of them responded to this topic with, "God is supposed to be omniscient, in which case He should already know what I need and when I need it and He could just take care of it." I felt like saying, "Of course, your highness!" Instead I responded, "Yes, but He doesn't know what you think about Him and if, or when, you want Him involved." When you pray, it not only invites Him into your circumstances, it also reveals how you feel about Him. It may show Him that you trust Him and that you believe He cares about you and is listening and powerful. Or it may show Him you are desperate or perhaps just trying Him out to see if He's really there and paying attention.

Whether it is your first step or one of many toward building a relationship, prayer is huge to God. It is what He seeks. **I believe He will make every effort to answer in a way that pleases you provided it is in accord with what is best for you AND for His kingdom.** Remember, you are not the only one in His kingdom. You may need to let go of your own very limited view of what is good in order to perceive how His answers are best for His whole kingdom, which although it does include you, does not ignore everyone else.

# For Guidance of Thoughts

When one hears the diagnosis cancer, it feels like a loud-speaker blaring "the house is on fire "or "the ship is going down." It doesn't take a genius in the crew to radio "Mayday," dial 911 or hit their knees; the "save my bacon" or "get rid of this cancer" prayers come easily. However, prayers that stop there don't give God a chance to participate in other arenas, such as your feelings, thoughts, and attitudes.

**Winning the battles in your heart, mind, and soul is not only important, but are often essential in order to win the war in your body.**

You need to give God access to them all. Remember you "are fighting a war on two fronts, one conventional and the other unconventional, with two adversaries, one you can see and one that you can't, one you can feel and measure called cancer and another you can only sense in the dark that I call the "Dragon." The doctors go after the malignancy that is attacking your body with weapons you can at least understand, like surgery, radiation, and chemicals, but those don't work against the Dragon. It is attaching your life and you are on your own. It wages a guerrilla-like psychological and spiritual warfare aimed at your heart, mind, and spirit. While it may not be able to kill you with weapons of guilt, doubt, fear, and anger, it can disable you enough so you cannot fight the cancer that can kill you."[3] God is the key. Prayer is essential. You don't need to face the Dragon alone.

Patient after patient has told me how much it means to invite the Lord into their thought life and how He has brought new perspectives, and with them, their attitudes have changed on their own. I can't remember their situations, but I do remember my own experience. Through the years I've prayed for all kinds of things, and often just that, material things. Then I would pray for my family, my agenda, my goals, maybe my friends, and eventually I might pray for understanding. Very rarely would I ever think to pray for help with my thoughts and feelings.

As I would read Scripture or look at the lives of people I admired, I realized they had ideas and feelings that I did not. My head and heart were just not there yet even though I wished they were. So, I started praying for the Lord to go to work on my thoughts: to order them, inform them, and change them.

To my amazement He has! Sometimes instantly, other times over weeks and months. Looking back, I can see that I have changed! I am astonished. I like it and I know it is His work in my heart, not mine. Attitudes are funny things. I often don't know where they come from, but I can readily recognize when they are a stumbling block.

Attitudes about what we expect and what we deserve in life are huge when dealing with cancer and can become major determinants of how we cope with the disease and its treatment. If your expectations are high and apart from God's promises, then your vulnerability to disappointment and grief are also. If disappointed expectations overwhelm you, you will be unable to focus on the plans and promises God has for you in spite of the disease and easily exhausted. I suggest you get God thoroughly involved. His work in this arena can be dramatic, rapid, and energizing.

One practical example that demonstrates how rapidly He can act is the whole arena of lust in men. It can be absent for years or it can spread like a prairie grass fire springing up wherever a spark alights. Some guys tell me, "Hey, window shopping ain't buying, so enjoy the looking." Those who want to avoid shopping for fear of stumbling upon an irresistible bargain have told me they pray instantly and have been amazed how rapidly the Lord can change their thoughts and throw cold water on the sparks. I would agree. If God is that attentive to such seemingly trivial daily thoughts, then He must be ever so much more concerned and helpful with every scary thought we can have about cancer and death. (Actually visual dalliances on the street corner or internet are not trivial, but you get my point.)

## GOD – THIS MAKES NO SENSE

When illness occurs or tragedy strikes, amid the turmoil of feelings, there is an attempt to make sense of what is happening. Why? Why me? Why now? What did I do wrong? What could I have done differently? Why is God allowing this to happen? Does He really love me? Is He punishing me? Those questions unresolved can become destructive feelings, some might say demons that can lurk in the shadows on the back roads of your mind with the dragon whispering all day and especially during the insomniac watches of the night, "Let me in, I want to occupy your thoughts and poison your attitudes."

Pray for protection from thoughts that conjure up guilt, shame, self-doubt, and fear. Fill your thoughts with what God is doing so as to leave no room for the demons. Using your "ammunition" and listening to praise music that is laced with God's promises helps. FM Christian radio stations broadcast around the clock and you would be astonished to hear how often the words of songs (often derived from scripture) will speak to you right where you are at.

Whatever their origin, be they spiritual or of our own making, the thought demons just love to bring up past wounds and get them festering. God wants to help with both. When you can identify such thoughts, take them to Jesus in prayer with confession and contrition and let Him wash them clean away.

Every time demonic thoughts steal into yours, start to pray. Remember Jesus is right there, whether you feel Him or not. It may seem like He is off snoozing on the job, but He is not. I suspect He is wondering, "Where is your faith? Will you remember that I am here?"

Stand strong and kick those thoughts out. If you can't, don't suffer or panic, ask for help. Read the narrative in Luke beginning at 8:22. Jesus and the disciples are in the boat crossing the Sea of Galilee. Jesus is sleeping in the bow when a squall comes up swamping them. The disciples, fearing for their lives, in panic, awaken Him. He rebukes the storm and turns to them, "Where is your faith?" At the same time shows them He is always with them.

Yes, He allowed the storm, even in the lives of the beloved twelve He was counting on to carry His message to every corner of the earth. Sure there were things the disciples could have done differently. After all, they were the fisherman, experts at sea, while Jesus was the carpenter's son. They could have taken two boats to distribute the load, found a more seaworthy boat, read the weather better, and so forth. Jesus let the storm happen, not to shame them, but to ask them one question, "Where is your faith?" I think it is fair to say that whatever the storm is in your life, the central issue is that same, "Where is your faith?" Will you remember He is always in the boat with you? Do you have experiential evidence that He is?

"Where is your faith?" is the question that can awaken us from our comfortable complacencies. It is one that fear, shame, and guilt would much rather never be asked. The Devil will do his best to distract us from it. These are normal feelings, neither right nor wrong, just real and the enemy will try to use them. The power we give them is under our control and is a measure of our faith. Be assured they don't come from God and you best steal your eyes away from them and focus your gaze on Jesus wherein lies the power to defeat them.

*God has a glorious plan for you. It is a plan that has no less potential and no less importance than it did for His first beloved disciples. It is a plan no less glorious in spite of the cancer and perhaps even grander because of it.*

## HOW TO PRAY: GIVE IT A TRY

Both learning to ride a bike and to pray have a lot in common. You can read about how to ride a bike, listen to instruction, walk all around the bike, and watch others doing it, but eventually you just have to get on and give it a go. It may not be pretty at first, but odds are you'll figure it out and get better with practice. That is the way it is with prayer. At some point, you have to just give it a go. There's no risk of skinning your knees or cracking your head, but the results may not be what or come when you expect.

Start with asking God to reveal Himself to you. If you know better who He is, then you will know better what to expect from His answers.

You can read about Him in the Bible, but what you really need to see is Him moving in your world. This might seem absurd if you are wondering, "I don't know if He is there, so I don't really want to pray to the oxygen in the room. To whom shall I pray if He is not there?" It's a conundrum. But sometimes you are in enough pain to do even seemingly unreasonable things.[4] So give prayer a try.

It isn't magic. There is not any one right way that works, but there are many wrong ways that don't. Apathetic, ho-hum, disbelieving prayers don't work. Take your lead from the Bible, then experiment and discover what works for you. There is no correct formula, but I can tell you my process now. I pray boldly, hopefully, and expectantly, and then I wait, watch, and listen.

I didn't start that way in the beginning. Once I got beyond just the big prayers from my foxholes while under fire, I began with small prayers asking for yes/no answers and sometimes the answers were just that clear. Other times the answer would come in events happening around me, opportunities/doors that would open or close, words spoken by friends or words of scripture that would jump of the page as if specifically written for me in just that moment. Other times, I would only get a leading as to which direction to move, though seldom actually words of instruction and never a complex sequence of instructions.

I think the best we can do is to try out the answers we perceive by acting into them. Always listening for more input and ever checking in our heart and spirit for that sense of peace that comes when acting in God's will or that sense of hesitation when we are not.

Prayer doesn't stop with the first asking. Listening, watching, and waiting for the answer is the often overlooked, but ever as important part. Listening for His voice, paying attention to what He is telling your prayer partners, and watching for answers in the events all around you.

Sometimes the answer is, "Ask again." Sometimes the process of asking again refines the real question making His real answer easier to recognize.

# HOW: REMEMBER WITH GRATITUDE

We know that the apostle Paul had some form of disability, a thorn in the flesh, perhaps impaired vision as a residual of the blinding light on the Damascus Road when he met the resurrected Jesus. It would be interesting if that were the case and would have implications for us. Paul was healed. He was given his sight back, but perhaps not completely, yet enough for God's purposes.

Why would that be? Why would Paul's (or your or my) healing ever be seemingly incomplete **according to man's standards.** Perhaps some remnant of that event was/is left as a constant reminder to him/us. We humans are so forgetful. Miraculous, thought-provoking things happen in our lives, even life-changing events for which we are immediately grateful, but so often our memory fades and gratitude slips away and any lesson is lost. Perhaps Paul was left with the reminder of God's work in his life and perhaps we are also. Perhaps that is a way to look upon our scars. Instead of lamenting them, perhaps we should be grateful for them. If their presence is a constant reminder of Christ's miraculous participation in our lives, we may remember to involve Him more quickly and confidently with our next challenge.

To this day, I vividly remember my first answered prayer or perhaps the first one I remember. It was pretty trivial in the scope of human events, but profound to me. I don't ever want to forget it so I have recounted it often. It propelled me to pray more often, although that was still infrequent until many more experiences were added to it.

It was junior year in high school, about a year after I had met the Lord at a Young Life camp. I had to give a twenty-minute presentation in front of our US history class which was filled with fellow football players and cute girls. I was shy, neither a star on the football field nor in the classroom, more of a mama's boy, slow to attain much manly stature and low in confidence. I had researched my speech topic completely, but just couldn't organize my thoughts enough to get them down on paper. I was to be sixteenth out of thirty which gave me plenty of time to suffer watching others do well or bomb and listen to other classmate responses which varied from wow, good job to poisonous snickers.

As my turn came, I had a dry mouth and a bellyache. Desperation inspired me to pray, "Lord, help me to do this thing. I know the stuff, I've done the preparation, but I'm scared to death, stuttering, stammering, knee knocking scared." Fear of shame does that. When called forward, a quivering blob of Jell-O rose from my chair and began to walk forward. Then something happened, the anxiety just disappeared! I turned, looked out, and began to speak. It all flowed. I was amazed and the grade was amazing. Whoa— God got my attention.

God had showed up just in the nick of time and unequivocally answered my prayer. It experientially validated what I had been hearing about Him. It became the first in my evidence list of answered prayers, a list that I have been adding to ever since. I no longer questioned whether God is listening or whether He will answer even trivial pleadings, but I had no clue I would have to learn to wait for answers; no idea that waiting was part of the prayer/trust dynamic at all.

I still dread public speaking and prepare aggressively but the fear is curiously tempered by a confidence that He will show up and equip me if I do my part. Curiously I have always had to wait for Him right up to the last minute. Then the trembling pulse in my chest and the sweat on my brow stop and it all flows. Speaking is not an area of innate giftedness, so it is always a blatant gift when it goes well and my experiential knowledge of Him grows!

When you're confident the answer has come, you've got to remember it. This is not as easy as it sounds. Life's events keep moving on and wash over today's answered prayers. Learning to pray, trust, and wait depends entirely on remembering.

**Boldness in praying,**
**confidence in trusting,**
**and endurance for waiting,**
**are only possible if one accumulates and remembers**
**the evidence of past answered prayers.**

Yet, many forget their answered prayers and then feel helpless when the crunch time of the next calamity comes. Some people keep a journal to record the answers to their prayers. Some make a pile of stones, one for each answered prayer. When friends gather we often recount the way the Lord has answered our prayers. It refreshes our memory, builds our confidence and encourages others.

**Pray Boldly, Hopefully, and Expectantly**
**Actively Listen, Watch, and Wait**
**Record, Recount, and Celebrate**

With remembering being so critical, I often wonder why our memories are so limited and erode so through the years. There must be something very important and very intentional about why God created us this way. Is it that the act of remembering and all it entails is so important to God; the effort, the focus, and the prioritization? Or is it that forgetting is fundamentally important to enable us to move beyond our wounds. Is it necessary to wash away some of the grit and grime of festering memories so we can heal? Perhaps it is a little of both.

Forgetfulness is an unavoidable default mechanism for us all; therefore, a habit of intentional remembering must be developed. For me, it is critical to remember who He is, what He has done and what He has plans to do. This requires regular review and regular concentration on Him. This is exactly what He wants— our attention. That is exactly what He needs to impart His truth, wisdom, and guidance.

## HOW: HONESTLY, HUMBLY, SINCERELY

If you want a real answer, every prayer must come from a place of humble honesty, not religiosity. This is not a time to be a puppet before some phony religious concoction of a god. That is not who He is or who He wants you to be. There is nothing wrong with sincerely reciting prayers written by another or praying scripture, but formality and correct form are not necessary. A sincere "help me, Lord" is all you need and is always heard.

The Lord has been lied to a million times, cajoled, stonewalled, cursed, insulted, demeaned, flattered, and bribed. None of it works. May as well get real or go home. He can handle anger. He has heard it before. He won't strike you with lightning for shooting straight. He knows you need to get it out and He is waiting with arms open like the loving Father He is, "Tell me what hurts so we can make it better."

My prayers started out pretty timid, but I found with each one momentum to try again increased. Initially, I was anxious as to whether God would show up, but that lessened every time He did. My process was slow because I so often failed to notice when He actually showed up and even then I often discounted His arrival as just good luck.

Some have told me they pray not because they really expect God to answer their prayers, but because they feel less lonely. It helps them get all their fears off their chest as if talking to God, even the God they don't really think exists, was a cheap, ever available, on demand, but passive therapist. I suppose it is okay to start there. It won't surprise God and it will at least give Him a chance to surprise you.

Others describe how all-alone cancer makes them feel even when surrounded by family and friends. They feel especially lonely during long worry-plagued, sleepless nights. They find comfort talking to a personal God, who they know is there, who knows their plight, and knows the rest of a bigger story.

It is the same comfort that the crying toddler feels after skinning his knee when swept up in his mother's arms. The knee isn't any better and mom isn't going to heal it instantly, but she knows the rest of the story and that's enough. It feels safe to the toddler to know that she knows and that means it's going to be okay. Remember when you held that sobbing child to your chest, that bitter sweetness. The sad empathy you felt for them was at the same time something wonderful for you— the way they came to you and clung to you. I'll bet God feels all that when we fall into His arms. Fall now. He is waiting.

## EXPECT A HEALTHY TENSION

Some things I ask of Him seem to be of such little significance that I wonder whether the perceived answer is really God or just a whim. Sometimes the issue will have no spiritual context and no way to be validated or refuted in scripture. So, I have been going with the answer I get. My hunch is that if there is any chance it is God, I'd better go with it and that trusting Him with what I think He is saying is not only the best I can do but also pleases Him. So I just do it.

Prayer for God's participation in decisions or dicey events does not relieve us of our responsibility to act in the moment as well. If there is no urgency, His expectation is for us to wait and hope confidently for His ultimate solution or provision. Otherwise, He calls us to participate in the process, while ever listening and watching for His leadership and intervention. He does not call us to passivity or to helpless sitting on our hands while waiting. Often we need to get moving in order for Him to guide our steps. However, we are never called to act independently in a way that leaves no room for His participation. If we behave as if we know the outcome already and that we will accept only our own best version of that outcome, then we have arrogantly taken over God's role and our prayers are only a sham.

Listening and watching for His answers are essential and must be followed by bold, trusting, and sometimes risky, and sometimes perplexing stepping-out in our best perceived direction of His lead. Inevitably there will be a tension between having the confidence He will participate while not knowing just when or how.

**There will always be a tension between having enough confidence to walk in the perceived direction of His leading, but enough uncertainty to keep us checking in for course corrections.**

It is this healthy tension between our actions and leaving room for God's actions that compels us into constant relationship with Him in the classroom of our lives so we will really get to know Him and this is exactly what He wants.

It is particularly easy to stop checking in when you think you understand the answer. I learned this lesson one morning on a hunting trip. Rising at five and grabbing a quick cup of coffee, we set out to wade the river and climb an adjacent peak for some pre-dawn scouting for elk. Five seasons and the last three days had left me with as yet no chance to even draw my bow let alone take a shot; hence an empty freezer. We were planning to travel light and move fast. As I left the tent, I wondered whether I should take my bow just in case, so I shot up a quick seemingly trivial prayer. I got what seemed to be a yes answer, so grabbing my bow and pack, I headed out wondering what God might have in store. I was hoping it might be a great encounter with the wily elk.

The others, packing only the requisite binoculars, moved off quickly through the steep timber and shale leaving me panting behind. Feeling bad about not keeping up, I was pushing my pace into overdrive when all of a sudden a breeze from my left brought the scent of elk, right at the 6400-foot level where I knew an elk trail threaded its way through the forest from an adjacent saddle where elk frequently bedded. I thought, "Wow, Lord, this must be Your plan." So I shifted into stealth mode and moved leftward scenting the breeze. An hour of effort rewarded me with fresh tracks, fresh scent, but no elk. My first thought was well maybe that wasn't the Lord answering my silly prayer, but my second was here He goes, doing it again, leading me into something entirely different than what I expect.

I had been moving slowly crunching nary a twig and stopping frequently to peer through the twilight for elk. Sometimes I would just sit and wait in the still darkness. It was a mature forest made up of large Douglas fir and Lodgepole pine, neither densely forested nor blanketed with underbrush, but carpeted with tall grasses, scattered wild flowers, and a dewy silence. The waning predawn glimmer seemed like an overture of the stars fading away to a gathering golden gloaming of the sunrise. It was awesome. I thought about my family, and I thought about my God. I thought about this book and the things I was trying to say, one of which is about the evolution of fear in our lives and in my life. Then I noticed something was different. Something had changed in me, which I discovered only in that moment. I wasn't afraid; I was loving a moment alone in the dark. That is big for me.

That visceral fear I'd had since childhood of being alone in the dark where there might be bears, cougars or wolves, a fear which I had prayed so often about, was gone. I can't say it will never come back, but at least in that moment it was gone and I was in the middle of an ethereal moment of fear free wonderment alone in the wilderness. I realized that if I hadn't shot up that silly prayer, "Lord, shall I take my bow?" I would never have had this precious experience nor would I be writing to you about how God will answer even the most trivial prayers. Maybe it wasn't Him at all, but He sure capitalized on it guiding at least my heart if not my steps as well.

I think God is saying "listen up" just like any father who wants to take his kids on an adventure. They can't imagine what is in store for them. They drag their feet and are about to whine when Dad says, "Trust me and I'll show you." God is saying that all the time and He will.

# IF YOU ARE FOLLOWING GOD, YOU BETTER PAY ATTENTION WHERE HE IS GOING

When I agreed to teach cancer medicine in a bush hospital in Ethiopia, I was skeptical, doubting that high-tech first world cancer medicine could have anything to offer a small third world hospital out in the bush next to the Project Mercy School. Once there and after feeling pretty useless for a week, I prayed, "Lord, what am I supposed to do here?" Then I seemed to get an answer, "Watch and pay attention, you will see."

Over the next several days, I noticed how often horse drawn carts brought in small women dying unable to deliver big babies days after their water had broken. For centuries women have been delivering babies with the help of a tribal midwife by just squatting in their "toockles," (single room huts: round, windowless, stick structures with conical grass roofs and walls plastered with cow dung). In that polygamist society, many young women are sold into matrimony as soon as they start to menstruate and soon find themselves pregnant. With immature pelvises too small for a baby to exit, both often die in childbirth.

That was it. It wasn't about cancer medicine at all. It was about teaching how a C-section (a relatively easy procedure to deliver a baby through the mother's belly wall instead of vaginally) could save lives— stuff I hadn't thought about since med school thirty years earlier and something that could be taught to the high school kids who arrived walking barefoot from hours away.

Teaching was fun, their attention intense, and the rewards immediate. The next day, one of the students brought his mother to the hospital thirty-six hours after breaking her water with her breach baby stuck in her pelvis. Now both are alive, and a pre-natal screening program has started at the hospital as well as regular teaching at the high school.

I learned a couple of things: ***God answers prayers, but sometimes you need to look around you to figure out what He means. You have got to listen first then walk into His leadings for Him to show you what He is up to.*** Just hang on and ride. I also learned if you teach the kids who are becoming literate, they will go home and teach their illiterate parents. An idea was spawned for new strategy for teaching health education to illiterate dispersed communities in the bush.

## Is It All a Story Problem

I suspect that sometimes the issue of our prayer is almost irrelevant to God even when it is huge to us. Perhaps it is just the "story problem" in a homework assignment to teach us the fundamentals of His relational mathematics. In school it was: Jim went to the store to buy apples. He had six dollars in change in his front pocket and $15 bills in his back pocket. Apples usually cost $6 per bushel. But it has been a dry year and apples are 10 percent smaller so they cost seven dollars per bushel. How many apples could Jim buy? The reason for solving the problem is for you and me to learn math. The real answer only matters to Jim and Jim is only a character in the story.

You and I are outside the story, but we need to know math to deal with life. What if real-life is in Heaven and you and I are like Jim in the midst of a story problem. We are dealing with the story of life with cancer: fatigue, cell growth rates, family dynamics, chemotherapy toxicities, work expectations, and cell kill percentages. The actual solution to our problems are irrelevant in eternity, but learning the process of dealing with them with God's help is tremendously important and of eternal significance.

A student can't get through life without learning the fundamentals of math, and we can't get into Heaven or run the Bell Lap well with without learning the fundamentals of walking with God. It starts with prayer and embracing those tensions that leads us to real health in the kingdom of God both now and beyond the divide.

# CHAPTER 10

# IS PRAYER A WASTE OF BREATH?

S ome have told me that prayer is futile. It is only a poultice for the desperate, foolhardy, and uneducated. I have responded flippantly, "It is easy to say it is impossible to fly until you have seen a bird or plane take to the air. But I have seen the plane (prayer) fly. It is true that it is impossible for you to fly unless you believe in flight enough to get on board." They respond, "Clever Doc, but it's not going to take me where I want to go!" To which I counter, "It just might. And if it doesn't, there are a lot of cool places it will take you, places you haven't been, places that at least a lot of others say are worth visiting. I know it is hard to get excited about visiting a place you've never seen, but if you don't like where you are right now, it could be worth a try. Think about it."

## MYSTERIOUS ANSWERS

Just when and how God will answer prayer for healing is a mystery. There's a lot more to health than just dealing with cancer. We all have issues, wounds, scars, and spiritual nutritional deficiencies. Jesus can bring healing to all of those and more. When He does we become stronger to biologically fight the cancer.

*Sometimes God intervenes in biological events to heal or alter the course of cancer and sometimes He does not. It is an unpredictable secret how he decides what to do and an even more mysterious why He sometimes changes His mind about what He is going to do. There is no formula, but there are some hints—one is for now and others are for later.*

## PERSEVERANCE

In 2 Kings, the twelfth book in the Old Testament is found the history of Hezekiah, king of Judah, the sixth century BC northern half of what is present-day Israel. Hezekiah had been the only king in Judah's history who remained faithful to God then he became ill to the point of death. The prophet Isaiah reported the Lord's instructions to Hezekiah, "Put your house in order, because you are going to die; you will not recover." Hezekiah wept bitterly and prayed, "Remember, Lord, how I have walked before you faithfully and with wholehearted devotion and have done what is good in your eyes." *The Lord responded, "I have heard your prayer and seen your tears; I will heal you... I will add fifteen years to your life"* (2 Kings 20:1-11). Hezekiah was blessed but eventually died.

**Over and over Jesus encourages us to be bold and persistent.** Jesus tells a parable about a man who awakens his friend at midnight to borrow three loaves of bread. At first he is rebuffed as all are in bed and the house is locked, but because of his perseverance and boldness, the neighbor gets up and provides all the bread needed. Jesus describes the point of His story. "Ask and it will be given you. For everyone who asks receives; he who seeks finds; and to him who knocks the door will be opened. Which of you fathers, if your son asks him for a fish, will give him a snake instead? Or if he asks for an egg will give him a scorpion? If you then, though you are evil, know how to give good gifts to your children, how much more will your Father in Heaven give the Holy Spirit to those who ask Him!" (Luke 11:6-11).

In another scriptural example the perseverance that is rewarded is not the nagging, bitter, self-centered sort, but a confident prayer for justice. In Luke 18:3, a judge is relentlessly pursued by a woman seeking fair treatment in a dispute with an adversary and he eventually grants it to her not because he is righteous but just to get her off his back. Jesus then makes the point, "Will not God bring about justice for his chosen ones (that he loves), who cry out to him day and night? I tell you, he will see that they get justice, and quickly." Then Jesus wonders whether He will ever see people with such a faith and confidence.

*Several times I've seen the Lord ostensibly change His mind. Whenever that has seemed to happen, it caught me by surprise. People in a virtually hopeless situation somehow had quality time added to their lives like Hezekiah. Sometimes tumors shrank inexplicably or just stopped growing, sometimes for months, sometimes years.*

What remained was always quality time in the life of a Windrunner who was living purposefully for God, who was faithful under duress. Like Hezekiah, a physical healing even if incomplete, gave them more time in this life, but not indefinitely. There have been cures too (remember Becky), but if they occurred in the setting of active treatment, we doctors usually try to take the credit, but there is probably more to the story than we know. In any event, when you think the show is over and God gives you a curtain call, pay attention; He has a reason.

*Isn't it curious that it was the Windrunners who had laid their lives so entirely in the Lord's hands who were at peace with whenever death might come, that were most often given extra time?*

Windrunners were the ones who had an eternal perspective and a special kind of perseverance. Not the kind one sees in a whining self-oriented "it's not fair" child. Rather, perseverance in pursuing God to discover what they could do for and with Him, instead of just what they wanted Him to do for them.

A good negotiator learns everything about what is important to the one sitting across the table and so does the Windrunner, but they do it not for the sake of exploitation or clever negotiation, rather so that in knowing God they will be better able to be part of what He is doing.

It seems clear that perseverance by the faithful in prayer will be rewarded. Why is that if God already knows exactly what we're going through and what we need? Why is the relentless pursuit of Him necessary? Surely it is to keep us in conversation with Him so that perhaps in the process we will really examine the issues, chisel them down to the core, and thereby understand both ourselves and His responses better.

*So the mystery is not whether we should pray or whether He will answer. It is not whether the answer will be good or whether we will receive what we really need. The mystery is what flavor of good and will we recognize it when it comes? It seems to me that in the passage from Luke Jesus' answer is clearly yes for them all. He is offering the ultimate good gift— a part of Himself, "the Holy Spirit to those who ask him," as if to say, He will give the definitive good gift, an indwelling powerful and all-knowing Spirit who will aid us achieve what we need, but even more importantly, help us understand what it is that we actually need most.*

If our children ask for all kinds of fanciful things, we often give them some of them purely as a gesture of our love. However, we generally engage them in conversation to help them understand what they really need and then give them that. I suspect that is what God is telling us here. He is trying to engage us in that very conversation. Therefore, we need to be persistent, but our expectation should be that He will help us understand what we really need and He will provide that. Sometimes I'll bet He throws in some of the other stuff of our dreams as well just because He loves us.

*This is a big deal to God. Notice in 1 Thessalonians 15:16 He says, "Be joyful always; pray continually!" Notice this is a command. It doesn't say, "When you feel like it," or "if you have time to spare." "Be joyful" isn't only for when things are going well; it is a command for all times and all circumstances. It is about things that are absolutely under our control: the attitudes of our hearts and the content of our choices.*

# DAY 1

# A WINDRUNNER'S JOURNAL

*I invite you to reread every sentence above which is **bold** and in **italics**. Write it down, in your own words if you wish, to remember it, reflect on it, discuss it, or even memorize it.*

_____

_____

_____

_____

_____

_____

_____

_____

_____

_____

_____

_____

_____

## IN HIS WILL

God invites us to pray, to ask, to be specific and be persistent, but "in His will." It is as if He invites us into His store, which He has stocked with the best things in life specific to our needs, which He understands better than we do. Then He says pick out and pray for what you desire and I will deliver it to you at the best possible time. He doesn't say select any store only His; not the corner ice cream shop where you can indulge every appetite.

Pray by quoting God's words in scripture (i.e. the Psalms), not to coerce or cajole Him into delivering, but to remind yourself of who God says He is and what He promises.

## IN YOUR ANGER AND CONFUSION

*God wants to hear more than our petitions; He wants to hear everything that is in our hearts. That includes our raw cries of fear, anger, confusion, and protests. We should bring them all before our covenant Lord and the psalmists provide us a model for how to do that.*

Those emotions are not to be bottled up, ignored or fixed. Hezekiah, ill to the point of death, "wept bitterly and lamented to the Lord that in the middle of my days I must depart" (Isaiah 38:3–10). Psalm 62:8 encourages, "Pour out your heart before him; God is a refuge for us," that we may be fully seen by God and we are "for you saw my affliction and knew the anguish of my soul. You have not given me into the hands of the enemy but have set my feet in a spacious place" (Psalm 31:7-8). He is saying to lay our problems on the workbench of His shop so that you and He, son and Father, can inspect them and work on them together.

> *Be merciful to me, Lord, for I am in distress; my eyes grow week with sorrow, my soul and body with grief. My life is consumed by anguish in my years by groaning; my strength fails because of my afflic- tion, and my bones grow weak.* (Psalm 31:9-10)

We have been given the Psalms as a script to pray and in so doing play our part in the drama of His kingdom unfolding. The psalmist's lament of the intrusion of death into life is not an invitation to self-pity or ingratitude, but an acknowledgment that the upward path while both difficult and treacherous, goes further: They are "God's way of reshaping our desires and per- ceptions so that they (we) learn to lament the right things and take joy in the right things."[5]

While a third of the book of Psalms is lament that seems to complain that God is forgetting His promises, the theological center of the book is that the Lord has bound Himself to a cove- nant of steadfast unfailing love that will be revealed in their ful- fillment. When we pray the Psalms, we are crawling into daddy's lap and pouring out the panoply of our emotions trusting He will respond within the context of His covenant and then resting in the hopeful expectation of that response.

"Many Christians don't seem to expect to suffer— assuming that if we are 'good Christians' who 'obey God's will,' we may face obstacles, but not great tragedies that seem senseless." The book of Job "shatters the myth that our own righteousness can protect us from unjust suffering."[6]

Job also brought every raw emotion to God— including his grief in protest in the face of suffering. He "does not confess lament as a sin against God, for it is not."[9] Spare yourself the question, "What did I do to deserve this?" There is no theology of retribution that suggests sufferers should look back over their lives in search of a secret sin that is causing their distress.

Harvard Divinity school educated theology professor J. Todd Billings, thirty-nine, father of two under the age of three, describes his response to the diagnosis of multiple myeloma and starting chemotherapy. *"It was not simple. At times I would cry out in grief to God; along with this, I would lament in protest to God for the sake of my young children. At times I would respond in gratitude for and awe of all of the gifts that God had already given, even if my life were not to be extended much longer... I found myself taking solace in these different yet complementary modes of praying and living before God: lament in grieving, praise, lament in protest, trust."[10]*

## LISTENING FOR ANSWERS

*Prayer is less about what you say than about what you hear in your heart. Most of the time it is like a transfusion into your bloodstream of a complete idea, no words necessary. Other times it is a word or a sentence downloaded to your brain. In my experience, audibly hearing God's voice is exceedingly rare. Sometimes, the message is vague and other time crystal clear. Those times were so astonishing that at first I wondered whether it was really God at all. Then I would answer my own question. "Who else could it be that gives me such sound advice?" Sometimes, it is a remarkably new idea or a solution I have never considered. Other times it is clearly not my first choice, second or third, so I know it is not me. Sometimes, it is something I can validate in Scripture, but many times I can't even find the topic in the Bible.*

My eldest son has schizophrenia and has many voices in his head several of which claim to be divine: angels, Jesus or God. Perhaps one of them is some of the time, but it is clear that most of the time they are not. For the most part they are controlling, frightening, defeating, and destructive leaving him bewildered and with no room for his own thoughts or anyone else's.

When most of us pray, we also hear voices clamoring in our heads or subtly nagging for our attention. They are the voices of self-interest, temptation, fear or fantasy which we can only recognize as fallacious once we have learned to recognize God's voice.

His words in Scripture help us to understand His character so that we might recognize Him when He speaks to us individually. "This is the confidence we have in approaching God: that if we ask anything according to his will, And if we know that He hears us— whatever we ask — we know that we have what we asked of Him" (1 John 5:14-15). ***To know how to pray, we need to know His will, and to do that we need to read the Bible regularly.***

It is true we can pray for anything we want. Sometimes He even changes His mind in response to one of our prayers, but He never changes His character or His will. One needs to know who God is and what He is about in order to direct one's prayers. In the Bible there are innumerable stories of Jesus at work in the lives of ordinary people, the crippled, the sick, the blind, and even the wrongdoers. Every time it looks different, but there are always common themes pointing in the same direction. These collectively are His will for mankind and exactly what we need to understand to orient our prayers and expectations.

# Day 2

# A Windrunner's Journal

*I invite you to reread every sentence above which is **bold** and in **italics.** Write it down, in your own words if you wish, to remember it, reflect on it, discuss it, or even memorize it.*

_____

_____

_____

_____

_____

_____

_____

_____

_____

_____

_____

_____

_____

_____

_____

## BARGAINING

Some try to cut a deal with God in their prayers offering their allegiance or some virtuous act in exchange for God granting their petition. I haven't come across any of God's words that suggest that is the way He operates or wants to be approached. Despite that "many religions urge people to give money to charity or to perform acts of generosity or community service to accompany their prayers at times of high uncertainty and anxiety. I would hope that neither the people who offer that advice nor those who follow it, believe that God can be so easily bribed."[8] *We are called to be charitable and to serve, but not as part of a negotiation. God can't be bought.*

There can be a blessing that comes with charitable giving and service, but it is not in a currency that we can exploit wherever we choose. It is not a chit that we can call in and apply to healing our cancer or buying our health. It can, however, be a blessing of the heart. It can bring the discovery of innate places in one's heart that wants to thrive on goodness, places that revel in connecting with the rest of mankind, and places so often hidden by layer upon layer of self-interest and charade.

Serving does more to give your prayers perspective than to buy answers. Wherever we invest our time and money, we soon discover our hearts are following. Perhaps tomorrow they will be leading. When our caring is invested in the poor and needy it is a good thing and one's heart can grow outward in goodness.

Give and serve, but be clear about why you're doing it and what you expect. It is not part of striking a deal for your health. I have never seen God bargain, at least not for your money or your health. There is only one exception; give Him your heart and He will give you all you need. That is for Him to know and for you to discover.

## GOD IN THE CORNERS

God does not live in the corners unless He has come there to rescue someone. When we find ourselves backed into a corner, it often seems there is only one way out; not so for Him. There is never just one way to achieve His goals for you. He is the God of the universe, so it is for us to be careful to not try to back Him into the corner with our own agenda. This seems to happen when the desire to follow Jesus shifts to predicting where He is going and leads us to get so far in front of Him that we actually lose sight of Him altogether.

It can look like this. Someone affirms their love for God and God's love for them. They seem to think that this gives them authority and stature with God. Then they divine a specific godly outcome for their situation. It is invariably a good one and consistent with some of God's past behavior in scripture and *incidentally favorable* to whatever their need might be.

*While God often responds in ways we expect there is a stumbling block: it is by His choosing not ours. When we expect Him respond in only one way (the one we have conceived), we back Him into corner and when we go looking there we don't find Him. Even worse is when a series of decisions are made based on certitude of God's predicted response. We miss seeing where God is really going and we find ourselves confused and alone in a corner with the consequences of our faulty decisions.*

A couple shared with me about where they believed God was leading them. They had prayed over the situation, both listened and watched for God's response. Some doors of opportunity had opened for them and seemed to affirm what they thought they heard God saying. They then announced the timetable they had established for God to complete what He seemed to be doing and they made commitments that were contingent on God delivering on both their expectations and their timetable. Whoa, that is putting God in a corner. It may all turn out fine and that may be exactly what God does, but I will be holding my breath. In my years of watching God move, it seems to me He doesn't like corners much and I will be surprised if He moves very often in a way so as to encourage these folks to put Him there.

The question then is: *Will they lose their faith in God or in their ability to listen and hear God's voice?* Or will they recognize that they had put Him in a corner by taking control of the timetable. God is in the business of teaching us about Himself and is careful not to mislead us. There may be some wisdom in leaving God some wiggle room. As creative as He is, He often chooses to meet our needs in ways and on schedules we have not yet imagined. Unless we are open to those, calamity may await us.

*It doesn't work to say to the Lord, "I will follow you," if you really mean, "I will follow you as long as you are going my way and on my schedule."*

## Naming It and Claiming It Puts God in a Corner

I met some faith-filled patients who were especially confident in their prayers. They counseled me that the best way to have prayers answered was to absolutely believe, not only that prayer will be answered, but how and then to claim it, and rest in peace waiting for just that to happen. When I read, "if you believe, you will receive" (Matthew 21:22) and "the prayer offered in faith will..." I could see part of where they were coming from but their confidence astonished and dismayed me..

Their confidence that God was going to come through for them in a particular way led them to spurn treatment for lymphoma and breast cancer. Some patients felt that taking therapy would reveal that their faith in God was inadequate or a sham. They believed with such a revelation, God would no longer come through for them. I must say I never saw that kind of thinking or believing work very well.

Their diseases progressed relentlessly just as one would have predicted for someone given no treatment. Even worse than disease progression was that beneath their spiritual arrogance and bravado was anxiety instead of peace and it destroyed the quality of their days, compromised the quality of their relationships, and left them totally confused when death came calling.

# Day 3

# A Windrunner's Journal

*I invite you to reread every sentence above which is **bold** and in **italics**. Write it down, in your own words if you wish, to remember it, reflect on it, discuss it, or even memorize it.*

_____

_____

_____

_____

_____

_____

_____

_____

_____

_____

_____

_____

_____

## ALICE: LOVING GOD DOESN'T EXEMPT YOU FROM DECEPTION

Alice was Adrianna's mother and Joel's wife. She came in pale, weak, and covered with bruises. It had all come on rapidly and just felt like "flu" until she started bleeding everywhere with teeth chattering chills and fever. Blood under the microscope showed Acute Lymphocytic Leukemia (ALL), with anemia and very few blood clotting or infection fighting cells. Her life was on the line and she needed urgent chemotherapy which is often curative in her situation.

Alice had **big faith**! Which to her meant she didn't need chemotherapy. Her church gathered around her and prayers flowed. Her pastor hovered over her as if to protect her from the medical staff and non-believers. He quoted verse after verse proclaiming God's power and ability to cure the infirmed and disabled and he extolled her as a mighty woman of faith who God would surely rescue.

She would quote Mathew 17:20 and Luke 17:6 professing all she needed was faith "as small as a mustard seed" which she surely had, and "nothing will be impossible" by which she meant nothing she could think of rather than nothing God intended. I offered chemotherapy as perhaps the means by which God would indeed cure her; after all sometimes He used a little spittle and sand to restore the sight of a blind man why not a few chemicals.

She wasn't buying that and was convinced God would do it "on His own" her way because she loved Him so.

Alice's daughter and husband weren't so sure. As she worsened every day, they pleaded with her first to take treatment and then tried to have those tender end-of-life conversations, but Alice would have none of that. She died, but before she died, she panicked. The end was full of pleading, anger, and disillusionment. It was not a good death. Adrianna and Joel were in shock. So much was left unsaid, a chance for cure was wasted. **God doesn't do corners**.

It seems to me, Alice took her confidence and belief one step too far when she extended it beyond the surety of God's answer to the surety of what that answer would be. It is hard for me to believe and to claim God will answer in the way I think best without leaving room for Him to answer in the way He knows to be best.

Alice's response was, "Why bother praying if He's going to do it His best way anyway." My sense is there are three reasons.

1) *He does sometimes change His mind and alter the natural course of human events after the fervent prayers of the faithful.* See 2 Kings 20:1–11 regarding Hezekiah; Jeremiah 18:7 regarding the nation of Israel; 1 Samuel 15 regarding Saul, and Jonah 3:10. Also, if changing the Lord's mind were not at least possible, Jesus would have known and would not have prayed in the garden of Gethsemane asking God to change His mind: "let this cup pass" (Matthew 26:39).

There is little evidence in my experience or in Scripture that God does that very often. He did not change His mind in response to Jesus' prayer because there was something bigger and more important going on. Knowing that, Jesus readily submitted. If God doesn't change His mind for us, we best submit and eagerly look for the bigger things to be revealed.

2) ***Prayer can recruit God's participation in circumstances where He might otherwise only be an observer.*** His participation may not involve changing the natural order of things, but it can change immensely how we experience them. Such a response from God is virtually certain if we are open to seeing it.

3) ***Engaging God in a conversation, praying and listening and praying some more gives us a chance to understand what His best way is, and to adjust our course to it enthusiastically instead of reluctantly.*** Understanding prevents us from wasting time and energy dashing down blind alleys before discovering "His way" by process of elimination.

Sometimes His way is dramatically different than my way. For me, adjusting to His course seems to also have three phases: knowing it, understanding it, and accepting it. Coming to know His will for me in a given situation may come first, but it doesn't come with enthusiasm. Then as I continue in prayer and meditation, perhaps over days, sometimes months, there often comes understanding, and with understanding comes acceptance, and only then can come enthusiasm. Somewhere along the line my course actually changes as a matter of choice rather than bitter resignation. It has been worthwhile praying even if I didn't get my own way; even if the natural circumstances don't change— because I have changed.

## BETTER BE READY FOR EVERY POSSIBLE ANSWER

*If God is in your life, He is working even if you can't see Him and your prayers don't seem to be effective. His answers are important even if you can't see them yet: keep looking. It is possible what He has for you does not have anything to do with cancer. While He didn't create the cancer, He is willing to use it to get your attention and get a conversation going about His agenda. If that is what He is doing, it is still up to you to pay attention and engage Him.*

You can still pray audaciously for what *you want*; He is the God of the impossible, but His focus will be on what **you need**. He can open doors and create opportunities you have never imagined. He can empower you in your gifts that have been sitting forgotten or unrecognized gathering dust in the attic of your aptitudes.

If you are bold enough, as a child of God should be, to pray audaciously, you better be ready to move out and act when the answer comes. So wait and watch vigilantly. As recorded in Joshua 10:13, the audacious and mighty leader of the Israelites, Joshua, faced overwhelming odds invading the Promised Land. Just as he had conquered Jericho with God's assistance, he prepared to attack the conjoined five armies of the Amorites. He prayed that the Lord would make the sun standstill to provide enough daylight for his battle to succeed and the God of the impossible answered. The sun stopped in the sky, night never came enabling Joshua's army to catch and decimate the Amorites.

I can imagine that when the sun stopped Joshua's troops, already battle-weary from fighting all day, may have been tempted to rest. However, once God answers a prayer, it is time to move right into the answer and trust God to guide and provide the resources. Joshua did and God did. The victory was astonishing. While Joshua could see the sun standing still, he still had to keep marching to discover God's provision of strength and stamina![8]

Conversely, the forgetful Israelites faltered when they came to the Promised Land the first time. Having just escaped from the Egyptians through the parted waters of the Red Sea and having witnessed countless miraculous answers to prayer in the desert, a guiding pillar of fire by night and the provision of manna and quail by day, they hesitated to cross the Jordan into the Promised Land for fear of the Canaanites who were so big. They had forgotten the size of their God: *"They still hadn't grasped that what seemed impossible for them to accomplish was exactly what God wanted accomplished for them."[5] They were not prepared and didn't move into God's provision and as a consequence got another forty years of wandering around the desert. If you don't like time in the desert, keep your eyes and ears open and be ready to move out when you start praying.*

# DAY 4

# A WINDRUNNER'S JOURNAL

*I invite you to reread every sentence above which is **bold** and in **italics**. Write it down, in your own words if you wish, to remember it, reflect on it, discuss it, or even memorize it.*

_____

_____

_____

_____

_____

_____

_____

_____

_____

_____

_____

_____

_____

## PRAYER MATTERS

God tells us to pray; we do so out of obedience. It should be no surprise there is a plethora of evidence that it matters. Anyone who prays regularly can provide countless examples.

My son Bryson was leading a pitch on the longest route up the tallest rock wall in the continental United States. The Yosemite Valley stretched out 1500 feet below and the top of El Capitan was out of sight 1400 feet above. Five days of climbing and sleeping in dangling hammocks had gotten them this far and five remained. He was about eighty vertical feet above his partners, on belay, lacing his climbing rope through various reusable titanium hooks, nuts and cams placed in whatever crack or tiny ledge in the rock he could find. While standing on a webbing ladder suspended from a quarter inch ledge, a "ping" of metal breaking free from granite shattered the silence and punctuated the beginning of a fall.

Would the next, a $50 piece of mountain hardware, placed with equal but tenuous care, hold? Would any of the others? The answer was *no* for the first, *no* for the second and third. Climbers die falling every year on this massif and the further you fall the faster you go and the greater the force on the next piece of gear meant to protect you ($E=MC^2$) and the greater the chance it will fail.

Accelerating into the void, Bryson watched with mounting terror as one after another pinged and popped out of the rock.

He described the cold, sweat-drenching relief when one finally held and he hung by his rope bouncing against the wall suspended above the valley floor. The *hallelujah* rush didn't last and was soon replaced by trembling and an invitation to panic.

Was it our prayers and God's intervention that got a piton to finally hold? We'll not know until later, but I will remain grateful and keep praying. Bryson tells us that it was only his refuge in prayer probably potentiated by the weeklong prayers of mother and father that rekindled enough composure to get him back on the rock to finish the climb. Prayer matters.

It matters for those we love and for their decisions and for the natural phenomena going on inside or around them. Bryson describes how fragile and thin the precarious edge of panic can be. I know that's true. I've been there. Again and again I've been thankful for a praying mother and a listening God. Bad stuff happens despite our best and most diligent efforts. Steel breaks free of granite. Accidents happen. Bears appear. Cancer kicks free the underpinnings of life. The question is what we will do with it. Will we panic and give up or will we pray.

It matters. Pray for yourself. Pray for those you love and recruit others to pray for you. Bombard God with prayer. He loves it. No illness, no injury or disability can diminish our ability to pray with intention and power and to make a difference in the lives of those we love.

Prayer was the principal motivation that got Fred going in his final days and weeks of life although that only meant awakening his heart and mind. ***Confined to bed, eyes often too tired to open, his days were still filled with purpose— praying for people, country, and causes. It was a purpose he could fulfill as well bedridden as he could any other time in his life.*** Actually better because there were fewer distractions and more time. That thought is a comfort to those like me who define our self-worth, albeit inaccurately, in terms of what we do instead of who we are.

There are many reasons for living in a community of God loving people, but prayer is a big one. Those who love you and know God's power will pray for you in times of need. I used to pray for suffering friends simply because God tells us to do so and because I didn't know what else to do. I often wondered whether my prayers really made a difference. An experience after a skiing accident crushed my face taught me how much the prayers of others matter. Too delirious in a narcotic haze to pray for myself, I was yet aware of a peace and assurance that must have come as God's response to a praying community of the faithful- many of whom I had never met. I was somehow nourished by their prayers to endure a very hard time with a strength that was clearly not my own. ***Prayer matters: Pray for yourself, pray for others and recruit others to pray for you.***

## NOW GO FIGURE IT OUT

Today, I awakened at five o'clock rehearsing a complex problem with several potential courses of action, each with serious consequence. I was submitting as fully as I was able to whatever God might say and listening intently for God's direction. I was pleading, "Just tell me what to do, what course to take," but sensed no answer. Minutes, then hours slid by and then I sensed, ***"I'm not going to tell you precisely what to do, but I'm going to give you guidelines: be kind, be loving, and be selfless. Now go figure it out. Just follow those and it will work out."*** It did!

## DELIGHT

There always have been experiences with the Lord described by writers that elicit the "you've got to be kidding" response of abject disbelief. I figure they must be a monk, a nun or somehow not in the world where I live. One such experience was the notion of continuous prayer that I mentioned earlier. Another was the repeated reference to "Delighting in the Lord." It sounded good, but I knew I wasn't there. Delight was not a frequent part of the experiential lexicon of my life. Then one morning while walking, I found myself lost in a prayer of gratitude expressing my delight in how God moves in my life: His provision, leadership, comfort, and His ever present intrigue. I stopped and thought, "Wow, I'm experiencing delight in the Lord. How cool is that, and I'm not even a monk. "

***Then I started wondering what had changed and realized that prayer had become a more frequent part of my life, a new***

*routine first thing in the morning and last thing at night. Many more times during the day prayer was inspired by mini-conundrums and eyes newly awakened to gratitude. It started when I crossed a threshold of certainty about Jesus being exactly who He claimed to be. It was no longer the "head" kind of certainty, but the deep down visceral "heart" kind that comes only from personal experience. Delight had not been a common experience for me perhaps because I'm a guy with limited emotional amplitude, but it is becoming so. It is no longer just when I am watching the antics of my kids or in the embrace of my sweetheart or skiing deep powder. It has found its way to the in-between times of daily life as well.*

## PRAYER FOR A SIGN

> *Then the Jews demanded of him* (Jesus), "What *miraculous sign can you show us to prove your authority to do all this?"* (John 2:18)

> *"What miraculous sign then will you give that we may see it and believe you? What will you do? Our forefathers ate manna in the desert; as it is written: 'He gave them bread from heaven to eat.'"* (John 6:30-31)

Jesus perform many miraculous signs during His life: turning water to wine, giving sight to the blind, healing the sick, making the lame walk, driving out demons, raising Lazarus and others from the dead, and on and on. Many on their faith journey today ask Jesus to give them a sign to help solidify what they want to believe. Others contend that God is no longer in the sign business; signs were for a different time 2000 years ago. Yet still others would assert that if you know how to read sign, you will see them often.

To read sign, you have to both know what you're looking for and where to look. With elk, it's not enough to just know what you are looking for: tracks, scent, scrapes, and scat. You have to know where and when to look: in the meadows at the forest edges at dawn, on steep shaded north-facing forested slopes during the heat of the day, and by the wallows as the shadows deepen at sunset. The first place to look for God is inside yourself, if you have ever granted Him access. Your heart and mind will tell you if you check the right instruments. Try measuring His presence with your anxiety meter, your confusion gauge, your solution index or your creative idea generator. That is where you will likely find Him.

Tracking elk is not successful every time. Even when you know they are about, there are signs you just plain miss. You must keep at it and it's the same with God. He'll be there and you just need to keep looking. With elk, it may be a subtle as an overturned mossy rock previously unperturbed for 100 years now displaced by an elk hoof. For us, God's work may be a subtle as an old troublesome attitude or worry now gone, or sleep now more peaceful, or patience now present where there was none—all kinds of things that easily go unnoticed or taken for granted. The signs will be there, but you have got to look.

Overt signs happen, too, but it's hard to know when to expect one or what to make of it when it happens. I remember when my brother-in-law, Buddy was knocked out and sustained multiple catastrophic injuries in a car accident. They had operated on his chest and abdomen and he lay totally unconscious and unresponsive on full life support with a fragile grasp on life. Unsure whether he would ever wake up let alone live, the whole family was struggling with the terrible question of whether to pull the plug and was pleading for a sign from God to guide our decision.

Even though he was unresponsive to everybody in every way including to painful stimuli, we explained to Buddy anyway the decision we were up against and asked him, if he was in there, to wiggle his right forefinger three times to let us know. Kind of an absurd and desperate request, but immediately without opening his eyes he wiggled his right forefinger three times and then about ten more for good measure. We took it as God's sign and left the plug in the wall.

That was the last meaningful wiggle or communication of any kind we could get from him for over a month. His coma was deep. We were left praying, waiting, and wondering whether the sign we had asked for and seemed to have received was real. Was it Buddy, was it God or was it a fluke. Had we saved our beloved Buddy only to get a rutabaga? Then all of a sudden he woke up— completely! Our wonderful old Buddy was back.

***God does sometimes give signs. There have been innumerable times I and others have asked and not recognized an answer, but there is no harm in asking.***

Some signs are hard to interpret and that must be the way, God intends it. My friend Bill was having a moment of deep spiritual reflection standing on the inner dock at the Young Life Malibu Club in Canada looking out over calm waters of Princess Louisa Inlet. He had been on a journey with Jesus for some time and was at a point of making a deeper commitment. He asked God to give him a sign to help him take the next step. Being an avid fisherman, he imagined that God's sign might be to have a large king salmon break water in front of him. But he no sooner finished asking for the sign and imagining God's response than a low-flying Seagull rewarded his plea with a generous fecal barrage that splattered across his face and chest.

I suppose there a lot of ways you could interpret that even if you agree with Bill that it came from God. Bill is a jokester without peer and he figures he got a sign. We know God has a sense of humor and Bill figures that God gave him a sign in a language that a comedian would understand. All I know is that Bill's faith has moved onward to a new level. Signs can be hard to interpret, but my sense is they are often very personal and don't need to be interpreted or validated by anyone else.

## Are We Supposed to Pray for Remission or Cure?

Yes, of course! God wants to hear from you; He wants to hear what is on your mind; He wants you to start the conversation and hopes you will let Him speak into it. Let your prayer be for a life that God designs: activities, encounters, timetable, and all. To do that you have to decide who your first love is: God or your life?

There is a time for Hezekiah-like boldness, but not right out of the gate. God already knows what you want. Now is a critical time when He gets to find out if you really care about what He wants for you. Start there: discern His will. "Okay, Lord, the script I was reading off of for my life has just gone blank. What would You have me do now?" Take whatever leading you perceive and pray for the courage and stamina to go after it. *Focus on His leading, scrap the bargaining, engage Him continuously, persevere on your knees, embrace the tension, and get ready for His answers.*

## Beware the Dragon

It may not be able to stop you from praying, but it is diabolically clever. The Dragon can derail your prayers by shifting their focus. Many who follow Jesus, tithe, and serve by loving others, but when it comes to the Bell Lap, their focus shifts to "all about me and my life." People who were living God filled lives of peace and purpose can be de-railed by Satan's ultimate tool, the fear of death—the fear of losing their secret love—their very own life. Peace retreats in the face of such apocalyptic fear and their prayers can shift from, "Lord, show me Your will for my life" to, "follow my agenda Lord and save it."

There's nothing wrong with wanting more life. God created it and called it good. It seems to me He gave it to us as a blessing, but with a purpose. It is not meant to be the end, but only a means to the end—an end that is enlightened and eternal and with Him. Heaven is another gift that those who show they love God more than life itself can count on. I am not so sure about everyone else.

We marvel at Daniel who braved the lion's den and the other Christians who died for their beliefs, eaten by lions, drawn and quartered or executed because they knew that their God is God, and life is only life. Had they valued their own lives unconditionally and in essence worshiped living rather than believing, then their words and actions would have been very different.

These events are not just curiosities in history nor just decisions made by past giants of the faith. A day will come for many of us when we will face the same questions. What will we do to preserve our own lives? Who will we ask for advice? Whose agenda will guide our decisions? The answers will determine the quality of our lives, and the presence or absence of peace. They will also determine how we run our Bell Laps. ***Those who have***

**really given their lives to Jesus know they are secure, and their salvation is secure; their Lord will be waiting for them at the finish line.**

## But He will ask:

*What did you do with the Bell Lap?*

*Did you run it with My Son or did you run it on your own?*

*Were you running toward Me at the finish line or away?*

*Did you pass the baton with all that I taught you or were you too busy with your own treatment agenda?*

*Did you focus your energies on grasping every day possible or did you lay aside worrying about that like Wendell?*

*Did you even give up the chance at a few more hours or days just so you could focus all your energy on the baton pass instead of probably futile salvage third or fourth line therapies?*

*Was My example enough?*

*Did you get it when I said, "Greater love has no one than this- that he lay down his life for his friends" (John 15:13)?*

When Jesus entered Jerusalem He knew what lay ahead. In essence His bell had rung. He did not hide or run away. He made every moment count: teaching, blessing, and loving to the very end; setting an example for us.

There are an infinite number of new treatments for incurable cancer. Treatment won't stop until we patients choose to stop; either on our own or when some compassionate, honest and perhaps eternally focused physician convinces us to stop. The best, most effective treatments are always used first. Every subsequent treatment is usually less effective and usually more toxic. Even when effective, most second and third line treatments produce shorter remissions than the one before with more consequences, less benefit. There are exceptions but they are rare, so always ask.

*Irrespective of the efficacy, any treatment can occupy the center stage of your life pushing all else to the wings.* To keep it out of the center takes constant energy and vigilance. It is a struggle for everyone. *Few, even the most committed and godly, are able to keep God on center stage, but those who do are the Windrunners. They all consider treatment and some take it very aggressively, some for years, but they are alert to when treatment will take more than it will give; they know when to stop or never start. They know because they pray; they ask God who is on center stage and they listen to what He has to say.*

Fear provides innumerable ways for deception to clamber back to center stage. Treatment always takes your time and physical energy. There are follow-up appointments, blood tests, scans, x-rays, and consultations. Then there is the travel and the waiting, and more waiting. More than that, treatment consumes your thoughts and emotions, not just to ponder your next treatment decision, but to fret about the results of all the upcoming tests. These are all legitimate, but they steal hours and days of your precious life and don't deserve center stage. That is exactly where the Dragon will try to put them.

*Thoughts about treatment and outcomes are inconsiderate.* They invade your consciousness whenever *they* choose; distracting you from special and otherwise joyful moments with family or friends, polluting your quiet contemplative moments, and worse—destroying your sleep. Just when you think you have all your questions and concerns addressed, anyone can ask how the treatment is going. WHAM! All the unknowns are back on center stage and you have to review them for your friends and deal with their reactions, their anxieties, and their fears as well. Whatever life is left can become tainted.

*It all boils down to prognosis. What is going to happen to your most precious possession, life, which the thief threatens to steal? The fear of losing it through death is the devil's favorite way to enslave you (Hebrews 2:14-16). The only solution is to give it up. Let it go, give it away to God and rest in His promises. Jesus tells us, "Whoever wants to save his life" whoever clings desperately to it, "will lose it." The devil twists his knife between your ribs letting the fear of losing life destroy it even while you still have it, "but whoever loses his life for me... will save it" (Matthew 16:25).*

That is precisely what I have seen happen again and again swelling the ranks of the walking dead. However, life worth living can return free of fear. If you let it go, it will come back better than before and without end, but you have to let go of one in order to grab onto the other.

*When you reach for God's hand, you step outside time.*
*You trust in His plan for you on this earth and the next; then He takes you there.*

You step into eternity and the pages of your story just keep turning; only He is writing the rest of it. Nothing more is there for you to worry about. As the prologue in this life ends, your eyes will close, the page will turn, and when they open, the real story will begin.

The Windrunners seem more alive than most because they are free and at peace. You can see it. They say in all sincerity, "I don't need to know whether the treatment will work or for how long. With God's help, I try to ignore Satan's whispers. I wake up each day and ask Jesus what He has planned for me secure in the knowledge that He is pleased with me as long as I'm moving toward Him whether I am on my feet, knees, or belly. I know one day I will awaken passing through the gates of heaven and that is all I need to know."

That peace and freedom is what I saw in Wendell, Fred, Chuck, Sallie, Ken, Connie, Dave, Larry, Gale, Bob and Alda, Doris and Al, Mary, Karina, and so many, many more. Some of them lived months, some years, and some are still living. All ran or are still running amazing Bell Laps with the wind at their backs, and under their wings, the Son in their faces reaching out their batons. Some have even gotten or are getting extra laps! Some are cured, but that is not God's first priority, so you had better not make it yours.

*Curiously this observer cannot recall any of the self-centered who became survival outliers and did extraordinarily better than their disease prognosis would predict. Whereas I can recall time and time again when someone who surrendered their timetable to Jesus seemed to outlive my expectations. Those who stepped outside time with the Lord somehow got more of it.*

# Day 5

# A Windrunner's Journal

*I invite you to reread every sentence above which is **bold** and in **italics**. Write it down, in your own words if you wish, to remember it, reflect on it, discuss it, or even memorize it.*

_____

_____

_____

_____

_____

_____

_____

_____

_____

_____

_____

_____

# Time to Write the Rest of Your Life's Script

When illness occurs or tragedy strikes, do you ask: Why? Why me? Why now? What did I do wrong? What could I have done differently? Why is God allowing this to happen? Does He really love me? Is He punishing me?

*Who is it that is really asking those questions?*

*After reading this chapter, how do you now think you should you deal with them?*

Read the narrative in Luke beginning at 8:22.

*What question did Jesus ask His disciples?*

*Why did He really ask them that question?*

*Is He asking you that question today in the midst of your storm?*

*How will you answer?*

**Boldness in praying, confidence in trusting, and endurance for waiting, are only possible if one accumulates and remembers the evidence of past answered prayers.**

Pray Boldly, Hopefully, and Expectantly
Actively Listen, Watch, and Wait
Record, Recount, and Celebrate

*God answers prayers, but sometimes you need to look around you to figure out what He means. You have got to listen first then walk into His leadings for Him to show you what He is up to.*

*What do you see God doing in your life today that is answering your prayers?*

# CHAPTER 11

# PRAYER FOR DIVINE HEALING

I f you believe your healing is just up to you and your doctors, then don't bother with this chapter. But if you're wondering:

> *If God might have a role in your healing?*
> *If He actually heals people in this modern age?*
> *If you have a role in appropriating His healing*
> *and what that might be?*
> *Why prayers for healing have not yet*
> *been answered?*

Then this chapter is for you because the answers to those quandaries are drawn from the scriptures, scholars, lessons from recorded history, and from the contemporary lives of patients.

Athletes exercise their muscles to run their Bell Laps, but the Windrunners pray.

After years of observing and participating in prayers for healing with my patients, I was introduced to *When God Doesn't Heal Now*[1] by Dr. Larry Keefauver, my editor, friend, and mentor. It authoritatively eclipses and expands on my own experience and has become the primary reference for this chapter. As a pastor and a theologian, Larry is able to elaborate on and contextualize what I, as a physician, have seen in my patients' lives. I have attempted to summarize his thoughts, sometimes paraphrasing them and other times directly quoting them. I would refer the reader directly to his book for greater depth, detail, and documentation.

**Scripture is unequivocal that Jesus is a healer. He heals out of mercy and compassion as it is in His very nature and intent.** Dr. Keefauver opens the Scriptures to reveal this absolute truth as demonstrated in both God's words and actions (Exodus 15:26, Luke 4:18, 1 Peter 2:21, Matthew 8:16, Matthew 9:35, Matthew 10:1).

God heals "every sickness and every disease among the people" (Matthew 14:36). Wherever He went "all who touched Him were healed" (Matthew 14:36). He gave the same power to His disciples "to heal all kinds of sickness and all kinds of disease" (Matthew 10:1), *but that was not the great commission.*

**It is clear that healing is for all and seeking it is His invitation**. Indeed, prayer is not suggested as an option, but as a command:

> *"For I know the plans I have for you,"* declares the LORD, *"plans to prosper you and not to harm you, plans to give you hope and a future. Then you will call on me and come and pray to me, and I will listen to you. You will seek me and find me when you seek me with all your heart.* (Jeremiah 29:11-13)

> *Is anyone of you sick? He should call the elders of the church to pray over him and anoint him with oil in the name of the Lord.* (James 5:14)

**Prayer brings us to the feet of Jesus to receive healing, but it does not dictate how or when Jesus will do that.**

Dr. Keefauver surveys forty-one examples of Jesus healing to show the relationship between faith and healing, and the simplicity of Jesus' methods: by a touch or a word, by being touched or by simply letting His healing flow. There was no elaborate ritual or stylized formula used or needed. Examination of the relationship between faith and Jesus' healing miracles reveals the critical need for our understanding of why He heals, when He heals, and who He heals. Only apprehension of that knowledge will yield the peace that comes with healing and dissipate the strife that accompanies the many myths about healing that have grown up both inside and outside the church.

Research of church history throughout the ages including the writings of Augustine, St. Francis, Martin Luther, John Wesley, and many in the twentieth century healing movement reveals, "**the undeniable truth: God is the God who heals, both in Scripture and throughout history, from the early church to the present day church.**" Dr. Keefauver has seen it. I have seen it in Becky and in others.

*However, what I've seen more often is a misguided fascination and confusion over divine healing which distracts individuals from pursuing God's primary goal for them; a genuine ongoing relationship with Him.* While the truth is that God heals completely those who trust Jesus as Lord and Savior, He doesn't always heal them completely in this life. If one's focus shifts from knowing God to negotiating one's healing now, you will miss out on much else of what God has for you now. Therefore, pursue God first, not your physical healing. Healing will come, maybe all or some now, maybe all or some more later. **One needs to be open to healing which is about a lot more than just the physical body. If it comes in time and space now, it is still only temporary.** Lazarus died eventually as has everyone else Jesus healed in the first century and ever since. *Ultimate healing is always in eternity.*

Healing of every malady in this life is always only temporary whether it be by our inherent immune systems, physician's medicines or divine interventions. Since the fall of Adam, life has clearly not been designed to last forever. So if you believe in a designer/creator God, then one must conclude there must be another purpose than life itself. Therefore, if the predominant focus of your life and your prayers is on staying alive, then your energies are misdirected and not aligned with the purposes of the designer/creator God.

It would seem that life is an opportunity to meet Jesus, discover our foibles and our desperate need for Him, get to know Him, then trust Him so profoundly that we can surrender every decision to Him, and experience the joy of running at His side on the unique race that He has set out a for each of us—especially on our Bell Laps.

His purpose is not solely about you and me. It extends to everyone, everywhere and it is our commission to share the knowledge we discover and the love we experience with whomever we encounter. **To the extent our focus on "staying alive" distracts us from His purposes we will have failed.** It is all about knowing, experiencing, and sharing Jesus. It is not about pursuing your own primary agenda: staying alive. It's not about building your faith or strengthening your belief so that you can negotiate with God and earn your healing. It's not about your agenda; it's about His.

# Day 1

# A Windrunner's Journal

*I invite you to reread every sentence above which is **bold** and in **italics**. Write it down, in your own words if you wish, to remember it, reflect on it, discuss it, or even memorize it.*

_____

_____

_____

_____

_____

_____

_____

_____

_____

_____

_____

_____

_____

# IS PROTECTION OR HEALING IN THIS LIFE A REWARD FOR FAITH?

*The fact that the twelve apostles were all willing to die hor-rible death young, and most did, is a testament not only to their having witnessed the risen Christ, but that long life is neither a reward for good works nor evidence of great faith nor a top pri-ority of God.* James was beheaded by King Herod Agrippa (Acts 12:2), Peter was crucified upside down in Rome fulfilling Jesus' prophecy (John 21:18), Matthew was martyred with a sword in Ethiopia, James, brother of Jesus, was thrown from the SE pinnacle of the temple then beaten to death, Bartholomew was flayed to death with a whip in Armenia, Andrew was crucified in Greece, Thomas speared in Italy, Matthias stoned and beheaded, Paul beheaded by Nero, and John survived being boiled in oil in Rome and was then sentenced to the mines on the prison island of Patmos and was the only apostle to die as an old man. Also Paul was never healed of the tormenting "thorn in the flesh."

God's purpose through them was not to brandish healthy specimens living long lives of physical vitality, safety, and good works. Nor did the people Jesus healed throughout the Bible become showpieces for His ministry. He didn't heal on a stage like some of the televangelists of today or encourage the afflicted to parade their healing. He said, "Get up, take up your mat, and go home" (Matthew 9:7). "Jesus warned them sternly, 'see that no one knows about this'" (Matthew 9:30). "See that you don't tell anyone" (Matthew 8:4).

Neither the Gospels nor Acts record wonderful things accomplished by healed individuals. Instead, they write about trials and tribulations purposed by God (James 1, Romans 5:3, 1 Peter 1:3).

## IS ANYTHING MORE IMPORTANT THAN HEALING?

***Jesus heals, but more significantly He saves***. He made that clear when the paraplegic was lowered through the roof. Jesus forgave his sins; He saved him. Then, so the crowd would know He had the power and authority to save, Jesus healed him (Luke 5:17–26, Matthew 9:1–8, Mark 2:1–12).

***Healing was secondary and only the vehicle for the message of salvation***. It was not because of the paraplegic's faith. Scripture says nothing of it, but the friends' faith made the healing possible. "When Jesus saw their faith, He said to the paralytic, 'Son, your sins are forgiven'" (Mark 2:15). Was Jesus rewarding their faith? Yes, but only incidentally. The main point is about salvation and not just of the paralytic. It all happened before a crowd so that the message might spread. If you are the one on the palate blessed with friends who will carry you in prayer to the feet of Jesus, just remember Jesus' first priority is salvation—yours and everyone around you.

# DAY 2

# A WINDRUNNER'S JOURNAL

*I invite you to reread every sentence above which is **bold** and in **italics**. Write it down, in your own words if you wish, to remember it, reflect on it, discuss it, or even memorize it.*

_____

_____

_____

_____

_____

_____

_____

_____

_____

_____

_____

_____

_____

# The Pursuit of Healing

There is nothing wrong with pursuing physical healing with God, just don't make it your primary focus. God doesn't.

There is a way to go about it and that starts with avoiding the stumbling blocks, those myths that so easily distract and confuse even the most ardent believer. **The greatest myth starts with if we believe, obey, and confess, He will heal.** There are several iterations of that myth that the Dragon uses to manipulate, exhaust, deceive, and to then defeat us:

- The key to my healing is my faith: great faith heals.
- If I stand fast in my faith, I will be physically healed in time and space.
- When I confess my healing I will be healed now.
- Prayer compels God to heal, but it must be the right prayer by the right person.
- Disease is God's punishment because of sin: unconfessed sin "finds us out" and manifests as sickness.
- In order to be healed, I must be touched by the right person.
- I can bargain with God for my healing: "If You heal me I will stop sinning, serve You, bring You glory, etc.".

Each takes some element of divine truth and extrapolates from it with a human twist shifting both the prerogative and the responsibility from the healer to the patient. This creates false expectations and, when unsuccessful, the potential for feelings of inadequacy and guilt. *"Myths about healing tempt us to believe that healing depends on us, on others or upon spiritual or religious rights and traditions. The truth is simply this: Healing rests solely within the sovereignty of God's Mercy."*[2]

# Day 3

# A Windrunner's Journal

*I invite you to reread every sentence above which is **bold** and in **italics**. Write it down, in your own words if you wish, to remember it, reflect on it, discuss it, or even memorize it.*

_____

_____

_____

_____

_____

_____

_____

_____

_____

_____

_____

_____

_____

_____

# WHAT GOOD IS FAITH WHEN I AM SICK?

*The truth is your faith moves God to save you (Romans 10:9–13, Ephesians 2:8) and in your salvation comes your healing. "But when you are healed, rest entirely on what the sovereign purposes of the healer are."*[3]

Standing fast in faith, trusting Jesus, does guarantee you will be healed eternally whether or not your healed physically now.

Confessing your belief in claiming your healing is neither a requisite measure of your great faith nor mechanism to obligate God to deliver on it.

Simple prayers by simple people can be as effective as elaborate prayers by special people who are quoting Scripture or speaking in tongues. It is the sincerity, vulnerability, and conviction of all these prayers that matters to God not the eloquence of the words or the credentials of those praying nor the invocation of a mystical spell or the theater of a magical incantation.

*Prayer opens the door for healing and faith helps us to receive and recognize it.*

While sin may hinder healing, God never punishes us by not healing. Rather He is always ready to forgive and heal.

Healing may flow through the laying on of hands, but a person's touch never heals; God does that.

# DAY 4

# A WINDRUNNER'S JOURNAL

*I invite you to reread every sentence above which is **bold** and in **italics**. Write it down, in your own words if you wish, to remember it, reflect on it, discuss it, or even memorize it.*

_____

_____

_____

_____

_____

_____

_____

_____

_____

_____

_____

_____

_____

# How to Recruit God into Your Healing

> *Is anyone of you sick? He should call the elders of*
> *the church to pray over him and anoint him with*
> *oil in the name of the Lord. And the prayer offered*
> *in faith will make the sick person well; the Lord*
> *will raise him up. If he has sinned, he will be for-*
> *given. Therefore confess your sins to each other and*
> *pray for each other so that you may be healed. The*
> *prayer of a righteous man is powerful and effective.*
> (James 5:14–16)

- ***Have others join their faith to yours in bringing your infirmity to Jesus.*** Don't go it alone. Surround yourself with praying friends. Ask the elders to anoint you with oil and pray for your healing and recruiting Jesus to gird you from any demonic attack and to break any personal bondage and any curse for sins of previous generations and your family.

- ***By faith be touched by Jesus – draw close to Him in corporate worship, praise, song and prayer.*** When you draw close to Him, He can reach out and touch you. The Dragon and Jesus are polar opposites. The closer you walk to Jesus the further you are from the Dragon. It will still be there, but its voice will diminish to the point of irrelevancy.

- *Submit yourself to the authority and will of Christ, trusting Him for your healing in His way, in His time.* The centurion's belief in Christ's authority made it possible for his servant to be healed from afar (Matthew 8:8). Mary and Martha believed in Jesus' authority when they sent Him word of their brother, Lazarus' illness, but constrained by their human agenda inside time and space with no concept of Christ's authority beyond it, they experienced untold grief for days waiting for Jesus to arrive. Their experience teaches us we need more than an understanding of His authority. We need to surrender to both His ways and His timing.

- *Believe on His words for your healing: "My words are medicine to all their flesh" (Proverbs 4:22 KJV).* "He (the Lord) sent forth his word and healed them; he rescued them from the grave" (Psalm 107:20). Bath yourself in God's words—not just His words of healing, but all His words. Read them, meditate them, listen and sing them and inhabit them.

- *Pray continually, persistently, expectantly with thanksgiving.* "Be anxious for nothing, but in everything by prayer and supplication, with thanksgiving let your requests be made known to God" (Philippians 4:6).

- *Praise Him* acknowledging who He is, who He has been and will forever be.

- **Wait patiently upon Him.** Cultivate your ability to wait by harvesting memories of all the times He has shown up for you and plant new opportunities—lots of little ones in daily prayer.

- *Obey the voice of the God who heals, His words in Scripture and His words spoken to you by His Spirit.* And obey even when circumstances seem to contradict His words by abandoning yourself and your pride to His will.

- *Repent and ask for His healing forgiveness.* Repent of past sins of omission and commission, for holding any offence against others and for any unforgiveness in your heart.

- *Expose every wound to God for healing.* Take every hurt and pain to Him and let Him bind them up and heal them.

- *Let God's light shine brightly in your life.* Seek God's glory in your healing. Let Christ use your weakness to demonstrate His strength to others – after all – it's not just about you.

*If you pursue the healer just for the healing, you have missed the point and will never find it. Pursue first the healer, not the healing and be assured the healing will come in a time and in a way that furthers the coming of His kingdom, both in you and all around you. Remember, it's all about the kingdom, and you are simply just a part of it.*

# Day 5

# A Windrunner's Journal

*I invite you to reread every sentence above which is **bold** and in **italics**. Write it down, in your own words if you wish, to remember it, reflect on it, discuss it, or even memorize it.*

_____

_____

_____

_____

_____

_____

_____

_____

_____

_____

_____

_____

_____

_____

# TIME TO WRITE THE REST OF YOUR LIFE'S SCRIPT

There are several iterations of that myth that the Dragon uses to manipulate, exhaust, deceive, and to then defeat us. Have you believed any of these myths? How has your belief now changed?

- *If I stand fast in my faith, I will be physically healed in time and space.*
- *When I confess my healing I will be healed now.*
- *Prayer compels God to heal, but it must be the right prayer by the right person.*
- *Disease is God's punishment because of sin: unconfessed sin "finds us out" and manifests as sickness.*
- *In order to be healed, I must be touched by the right person.*
- *I can bargain with God for my healing: "If You heal me I will stop sinning, serve You, bring You glory, etc."*

**"Myths about healing tempt us to believe that healing depends on us, on others or upon spiritual or religious rights and traditions. The truth is simply this: "Healing rests solely within the sovereignty of God's Mercy."[2]**

*Have you believed any of these myths?*

*How has your belief now changed?*

Use this as a checklist as you pray for your divine healing:

☐ Have others join their faith to yours in bringing your infirmity to Jesus.

☐ By faith be touched by Jesus—draw close to Him in corporate worship, praise, song, and prayer.

☐ Submit yourself to the authority and will of Christ, trusting Him for your healing in His way, in His time.

☐ Bathe yourself in God's words—not just His words of healing, but all His words. Read them, meditate them, listen, sing them, and inhabit them.

☐ Pray continually, persistently, expectantly with thanksgiving.

☐ Praise Him acknowledging who He is, who He has been and will forever be.

☐ Wait patiently upon Him. Cultivate your ability to wait by harvesting memories.

☐ Obey the voice of the God who heals, His words in Scripture, and His words spoken to you by His Spirit.

☐ Repent and ask for His healing forgiveness. Expose every wound to God for healing. Let God's light shine brightly in your life.

# CHAPTER 12

# A PLACE CALLED PEACE

*Through the heartfelt mercies of our God, God's sunrise will break in upon us, shining on those in darkness, those sitting in the shadow of death... then showing us the way, one foot at a time down the path of peace.* (Luke 1:78-79 MSG)

Many in life sense something is missing. A cancer diagnosis is the experience of the utter darkness in the shadow of death, the unequivocal absence of peace, and a yearning for the light while there is still time to do something about it.

*Do not be anxious about anything, but in every situation, by prayer and petition, with thanksgiving, present your requests to God. And the peace of God, which transcends all understanding, will guard your hearts and your minds in Christ Jesus.* (Philippians 4:6-7)

*This is what the* LORD *says*—your Redeemer, the Holy One of Israel: *"I am the* LORD *your* God, *who teaches you what is best for you, who directs you in the way you should go.* **If only you had paid attention to my commands, your peace would have been like a river, your well-being** like the waves of the sea. (Isaiah 48:17-18 emphasis added)

**Peace comes from the union of man, once estranged from God, now reunited with Him: "His law is love and His gospel is peace."**[1]

Many of us have been or still are hypocrites, myself included. What we say we believe must only be fantasies, belied by who we are and how we act. It is all subconscious because we aren't paying attention to the disconnect. However, we find out who we really are when the Bell rings and our life is on the line—and so does the rest of the world. What a person really thinks spills out of their soul into their behavior when stress strikes and that is what makes history!

When words and actions are not congruent, people notice. When peace is nowhere to be found, we struggle and wonder why and people notice. It doesn't matter much unless it drives them away from either us or the truth. It hurts the hypocrite the most. If you are one, public opinion probably matters to you, so you best sort your act out, and in the process you may stumble on the road to real peace.

*Peace is a place where joy is the air you breathe.* **It is rather like a suburb of Heaven, a dwelling place next door to Jesus where you get to connect with Him often. Those who find it know when they have arrived and they want to stay, but life moves on. New issues emerge to distract and soon they discover they are no longer in Peace and must go searching again. Fortunately, having been there once, it is easier to find the way back.** Eventually they learn not to stray from Jesus' side, or at least not beyond the reach of His voice. The key to living in Peace is knowing His wisdom can be trusted and regularly seeking it until it becomes your very life blood—that which powers every brain cell to think and every muscle to act.

# DAY 1

# A WINDRUNNER'S JOURNAL

*I invite you to reread every sentence above which is **bold** and in **italics**. Write it down, in your own words if you wish, to remember it, reflect on it, discuss it, or even memorize it.*

_____

_____

_____

_____

_____

_____

_____

_____

_____

_____

_____

_____

_____

## WHAT'S IT LIKE?

I have witnessed peace in the eyes, words, and actions of Windrunners and I've experienced it amidst some of the greatest stresses of my life, but only in the last few years. As hokey as it sounds, I felt it come over me when I heard His voice, "Wait and trust," as I faced the grizzly bear on the mountainside. A decade later, I experienced it again while I was broken and bleeding, first in an ambulance and later in an ICU. A high speed collision with another skier impaled his helmet into my face with crushing force. Rendered helpless, weak from blood loss, and virtually blind by the fractures and swelling, I felt an unearthly assurance of being in God's arms and that everything would be all right, even though I could not have defined what "all right" would be.

*It must have been the mercy of God potentiated by prayers of people I know and others I have never met that brought so much comfort. I can't say the suffering lessoned as it was far beyond the scope of my experience, yet endurance was surely fortified.*

I don't remember fearing the outcome; it would be just as it should be. I did not fear that my body and spirit would stray from God's grasp; it would be sufficient for the task at hand. It was still lots of blood and lots of awful, yet peaceful.

## WHAT PEACE DOESN'T DO

I did learn something new about peace. It didn't inspire passivity or helplessness either with the bear or the medics. I still felt very much engaged in the events around me and the decisions that needed making, but it seemed that the peace precluded panic. Without disabling fear, intense focus on the problems at hand was possible. I recall telling a medic, "I don't mind if I'm going to die because I'm excited about going to Heaven, but if I'm not dying, don't screw this up, do X, don't do Y, and beware of Z."

*I don't believe God sends us peace so we can abdicate our responsibilities to care for ourselves, but rather to give us the coherence to do just that and do it well.*

Trusting in God's goodness and ultimate provision does not mean sitting on your hands, disengaging your brain or becoming passive, nor does it mean extending that same trust to everyone else, doctors included. They are not God's puppets. While God could control their every move, He won't. They are still free to make mistakes. We must remain fully engaged with the gifts of discernment God has given us. Keep an eye on them. Question them and pray for them.

David trusted God, but he took his giftedness with a slingshot along when he faced Goliath. Jesus used His wits, wisdom, and words when confronting the Pharisees. He knew better than anyone of God's power and plan, but He had a role to play and so do you. Use your intellect, voice, and assertiveness, but under His direction. Pray your way into it, listen for His guidance, and wait for the peace that He will send to validate and enable the direction in which you're moving.

# DAY 2

# A WINDRUNNER'S JOURNAL

*I invite you to reread every sentence above which is **bold** and in **italics**. Write it down, in your own words if you wish, to remember it, reflect on it, discuss it, or even memorize it.*

_____

_____

_____

_____

_____

_____

_____

_____

_____

_____

_____

## You Can't Fake Peace

*Peace is not about what you do or how you look, but what you know which determines how you feel. It may look many ways, but it feels always the same. Peace is full of comfort, confidence, purpose, and destiny. Uncertainty doesn't evaporate, but it does move into the background where it can't be in control.*

If amid the chaos of your life you're not experiencing peace, it may be telling you something about the direction you're going, the decisions you are making, who you are listening to, and perhaps the true depth of your faith.

However, don't get misguided expectations of your faith and its peace. It is true that when they arrive in full bloom, terror will depart and take with it worry, but misery, hassle, disappointment, pain, and some uncertainties may remain. They are the unavoidable fabric of human existence. The presence of a faithful God and His peace will enable you to endure them, possibly overcome, but never eradicate. That is for later, when we cross the divide, move next door to Heaven and stand next to Jesus.

## Joyless Christians

Modern, educated, and even skeptical people may be drawn to Christianity because it gives them a language and a community to express moral beliefs they otherwise already have on strictly secular grounds. However, such religiosity does not produce the fruit of the Spirit: love, peace, and joy.

*The annals of good Christians battling cancer are bursting at the seams with joyless people. They may love God.* They may seek God. They may even serve God with every precious ounce of their energy, but despite it all, and despite God's promises of love, purpose, and Heaven, joy escapes them. Even the *pretend joy* that masquerades as *real joy* has evaporated. It is not their fault. They are good, but they lack trust. The deceit of a demon has convinced them that belief was enough and that stepping out in risk with trust was not necessary.

*The demon whispers that being a good person with dedication and discipline is enough, but joy does not follow. It is not an emotion you can choose or earn. Joy is a gift like peace that comes only when you have trusted Jesus enough times that trust has become the quintessential characteristic of your relationship such that the Holy Spirit inhabits you and leads you on. Then peace and joy happen. Without such trust, no amount of worship or faithful service will create them. Against such trust no demon can prevail.*

# DAY 3

# A WINDRUNNER'S JOURNAL

*I invite you to reread every sentence above which is **bold** and in **italics**. Write it down, in your own words if you wish, to remember it, reflect on it, discuss it, or even memorize it.*

_____

_____

_____

_____

_____

_____

_____

_____

_____

_____

_____

_____

_____

## Only Absence Defines Real Presence

*Can we learn the value and power of love without experiencing its absence?*

*Can we know the bliss of security without experiencing the risk of living without it?*

*Are we given free will and a semblance of control in this life that we might experience their limitations?*

Neither free will or control guarantees security nor produces peace, but we clamber after both. Perhaps we need to experience their charade to discover that something is missing. Cancer is the anvil on which the charade crumbles. Windrunners figured that out.

## The Place Windrunners Live

**The first word that came to mind when I met the Windrunners was "peace."** They seemed to live in a place that I could only visit now and then. Despite the trauma of their circumstances they somehow lived on a plane beyond the reach of the Dragon.

**Peace seemed to be an ingredient in producing better responses to therapy rather than the other way around.** Response to therapy produces only the briefest sensation of peace because response does not defeat fear, only God can do that.

I suspect the peace that Windrunners were experiencing was a taste of what enabled Jesus to endure the scourging and the cross. Perhaps we too must face our own cross-like suffering to experience that peace and tap into God's vast wealth of mercy and grace and to finally know that it is real. *Once experienced, such peace is never forgotten and begets a strength that is never lost and with it understanding and gratitude. It prepares one for greater peril, even to look boldly into the face of death, and with Paul taunt, "Where O death is your victory? Where, O death is your sting?" (1 Corinthians 15:55). You know it's gone and you will never be the same.*

# DAY 4

# A WINDRUNNER'S JOURNAL

*I invite you to reread every sentence above which is **bold** and in **italics**. Write it down, in your own words if you wish, to remember it, reflect on it, discuss it, or even memorize it.*

_____

_____

_____

_____

_____

_____

_____

_____

_____

_____

_____

_____

_____

## PEACE IS A GIFT, BUT NOT A REWARD

Some think that if you are living in the middle of God's will, bad things will not happen. That is a myth. Jesus was in the boat with the disciples on the Sea of Galilee when the squall struck threatening to capsize and drown them. He is always in our boats when the storms strike and He is not worried. He knows how our stories will end and He is waiting for us to notice that He is there and to engage Him (Mark 4:36-38).

The apostle Paul knew this when he wrote to the imperiled Christians at Thessalonica. "All this trouble is a clear sign that God has decided to make you fit for his kingdom. You are suffering but justice is on the way" (2 Thessalonians 1:5 MSG). So it may be with the challenges we each face. When you examine yours look for traces of God's tutelage and then walk into them boldly and be encouraged. *He is with you. "If your life honors the name of Jesus, he will honor you" (2 Thessalonians 1:11-12 MSG) and make you fit to meet His calling. Let your pain drive you into His purpose.*

*Authenticity can emerge when you trust God for the ultimate outcome of your life and that makes posing and lying in order to manipulate the outcome you fear all unnecessary. Think about that for a minute. Do you fear the life you might live if all you have got is the real you? God doesn't!*

When the rich tapestry of life is unraveling, the trappings of success are fading and the promises of earthly tomorrows vanishing, the conditions for a deepening relationship with Jesus are never better and the origins of the peace He brings never clearer. "Blessed are the poor in spirit." "You're blessed when you're at the end of your rope. With less of you there is more of God and his rule" (Matthew 5:4, NIV/ MSG)

# DAY 5

# A WINDRUNNER'S JOURNAL

*I invite you to reread every sentence above which is **bold** and in **italics**. Write it down, in your own words if you wish, to remember it, reflect on it, discuss it, or even memorize it.*

_____

_____

_____

_____

_____

_____

_____

_____

_____

_____

_____

_____

_____

# Time to Write the Rest of Your Life's Script

*I don't believe God sends us peace
so we can abdicate our responsibilities to care for ourselves,
but rather to give us the coherence to do just that and
do it well.*

Trusting in God's goodness and ultimate provision does not mean sitting on your hands, disengaging your brain or becoming passive, nor does it mean extending that same trust to everyone else, doctors included. Here are the steps for you to follow:

Pray your way into it.

Listen for His guidance.

Wait for the peace that He will send to validate
and enable the direction in which you're moving.

If amid the chaos of your life you're not experiencing peace, it may be telling you something about the direction you're going, the decisions you are making, who you are listening to, and perhaps the true depth of your faith.

*Pray and ask the Lord to reveal to you if there is something in the direction you are going that needs changing.*

*Ask Him if the decisions you are making are in line with His plan for you.*

*Think carefully about who you are listening to and ask the Lord to reveal those who are deceiving you and distracting you from His truth.*

# CHAPTER 13

# BACKSTRETCH WORK FOR WINDRUNNERS

"Sometimes *God permits what he hates, to accomplish that which He loves.*" - Joni Eareckson Tada[1]

"*Blessed are the poor in spirit.*" (Mathew 5:3)

"*Choosing to live as if you are dying creates the optimal conditions for your soul to mature.*" – Unknown[2]

T he backstretch starts as soon as there is evidence that treatment is working, a partial remission (50 percent shrinkage), complete remission (100 percent disappearance), or completion of treatment with hope for cure. That doesn't mean all the fears and concerns encountered in the near corner that we talked about in *Cancer's Bell Lap and the Dragon Behind the Door* are gone. The Dragon is still there, just not as close. You still have to deal with and overcome them all because until you do, the Dragon will creep up on you when you least expect it.

The beginnings of remission free up some room on the workbenches of our mind and heart to engage some new ideas or pull ones off the back shelves where they have been gathering dust. Completing the challenges presented in the first corner and engaging the new ones in this chapter are worthwhile for many reasons, but one is that it erases many worries, refreshes life, and maybe lengthens it. "Some studies show that worry and stress can actually increase the risk of relapse" (*After Cancer Care*, p. 31). They warrant attack on all fronts and by all means. Treat yourself to counseling and engage the wonderful counselor. Each of us can use all the help we can get. Only the proud and arrogant don't recognize that.

***God wants to do great things with you from the platform of your suffering.*** He knows you are not okay and He wants you to know it is okay to not be okay. When you recognize that, it is the beginning of walking into the blessing He has for you. He wants to bestow divine favor on you in the midst of it. Even as it entails some homework on your part, it will bring you joy. It starts now and it doesn't hurt.

***God is not done with you yet***. Here's the good news: running your Bell Lap well is not about trying ever harder to achieve greatness and polish your legacy, but rather it is about letting God have His way with you, letting Him lead you into the destiny He has already planned and prepared for you. You just need to show up, pay attention, and respond daily, moment by moment.

Joni Earekson Tada began her Bell Lap when a nearly fatal diving accident rendered her quadriplegic and wheelchair bound in her teens. She recalls now that when she was struggling with a depression she didn't want, despondent over what God had permitted, and fearing what He might permit next, a friend, Steve Estes told her, "Sometimes God permits what He hates to accomplish what He loves." Joni now reports from her wheelchair that her suffering has, "made her faith life more muscular...deepened her prayer life...expanded her interest in reading the Bible and has grown her character by building patience and endurance,"[1] all of which has bolstered Joni's confidence that God hates suffering. He has lovingly nurtured and carried her through it. With God's help, she has reinvented her life: getting married, painting with a brush in her teeth, writing, singing, and speaking out through the pain of her own struggles including cancer to share the hope and love of Christ to all of us, particularly the disabled, underprivileged, and afflicted.

***Breathe a sigh of relief. God does not measure greatness as the world does by quantitating achievements, wealth, influence, or status. Those are all fine when they come by His blessing, but***

*none are as precious to Him as introducing a granddaughter to Jesus or simply living a life of confidence and peace holding on to His hand. God has a purpose for you wherever you are, even on a physical decrescendo. There are things you can do, ways you can be, words you can utter. He has prepared them in advance for you. You don't need to dream them up; He will bring them to you if the eyes of your heart are open to receive them. He will orchestrate the last chapters of your life and reveal your destiny.*

# DAY 1

# A WINDRUNNER'S JOURNAL

*I invite you to reread every sentence above which is **bold** and in **italics.** Write it down, in your own words if you wish, to remember it, reflect on it, discuss it, or even memorize it.*

_____

_____

_____

_____

_____

_____

_____

_____

_____

_____

_____

_____

## KNOWING YOURSELF

The best backstretch starts with knowing yourself. Until you understand your own story and everyone in it, you cannot make peace with it or them. "Our story begins with the characters who gave us birth including their past relationships with their parents and their issues such as success and shame; power and abuse; love, loss and addiction; heartache and secrets; and family myths."[3] Before that, it began with the God who made you in His image. Getting to know who He is, is the beginning of discovering who you are. Only the real you can participate in His good plans for the endgame.

*Until you have accepted God's grace and lavished it on your past, you may find it difficult to anticipate it in your future or to lavish it on anyone else. The deeper the hurt and sorrow of life the more likely one is to crumple to their knees before Jesus, the very place where you get to know Him best. Are you there yet? It's only a two-foot drop.*

You are His chosen and not because of what you can do. Yet what you do with His help helps you understand who He is. Getting to know Him is the silver lining in the clouds that suffering brings. He will show you what you have to offer and empower you with the passion to offer it. He wants to use you to help usher in His kingdom.

Before you can bless others, you need to receive your own blessing. A good place to start would be to read Henry Nouwen's, *Life of the Beloved*. It is short, only 149 pages. You will be blessed. Get it now.

# Day 2

# A Windrunner's Journal

*I invite you to reread every sentence above which is **bold** and in **italics**. Write it down, in your own words if you wish, to remember it, reflect on it, discuss it, or even memorize it.*

_____

_____

_____

_____

_____

_____

_____

_____

_____

_____

_____

_____

# DISCOVERING YOUR OWN BLESSEDNESS

*The power to bless others comes from a profound sense of your own blessedness which can produce a wellspring of gratitude in your heart.* We don't always feel that, but God wants us to. We are His beloved despite all our mistakes and broken pieces. Looking back to your parents' and grandparents' lives, you may find where some of your broken pieces came from.

Discover the message of the pieces, the good, bad and even the ugly, that were the primordial soup out of which you became you. Then examine your decisions and the decisions of the others that affected you. Bring it all before the Lord and invite Him to sift through it all and guide you to make peace with it. Let Him teach you how to forgive yourself as well as how to forgive those who let you down. Then let Him support you in letting go and leaving behind the bits and pieces for which there is no explanation. Let Him heal your stuff and give you enough understanding and grace so that you can pass on a healthy baton.

Pray for His forgiveness, "Lord, forgive us our trespasses," and **then receive it**. Keep praying until you do. Then you can fulfill the commission that follows in the Lord's Prayer: "Lord, forgive us our trespasses **as we forgive others**." Every one of our unhealed wounds and every forgiveness we do not grant burdens the next generation. We cannot change our past, but we can make peace with it and learn from it so that it will not corrupt the rest of our future or that of our loved ones. Even the worst or seemingly worthless among us has a story to tell which someone needs to hear and may well help them put the pieces of their life together better.

*Get intentional. Use some of those otherwise wasted moments driving down the road or sitting in doctors' offices to dig into the attic of your mind where memories have been gathering dust for years as you have been dealing with the roller coasters of life. Process those memories with others and with God. Celebrate the good and draw lessons from the bad. If you have no one to do that with, invite God to come along to digest them with you as you record them in a journal. Remember the Lord doesn't collect or record the bad stuff; He forgives it and forgets it.*

Your written thoughts need no beginning or end. Just start and they will lead you as the padlock comes off of your memories and secrets. You may be astounded at how thoughts and feelings that you didn't even know you had will come tumbling out and how, with the Lord's wisdom and grace, start making more sense.

You are the only expert on your life so there's no reason to feel inadequate in describing it. Write about the people you have loved and why; the places you've lived and how they affected you; and the things that made you laugh, cry and tremble. Add your trials, your disappointments and your triumphs. Relive it all and listen to what your life is telling you. Permit yourself to be surprised as the details you have long forgotten start appearing on the page. Some of the conclusions may even warrant passing on with your baton.

You needn't write it for others to read or else you might create a charade of posing and braggadocio. It is most meaningful if you are raw, real, and humble, all of which you can do best in private. Then it might be worth leaving to a loved one(s) if you're unable to deliver it all in person or if they are still too young to receive it; decide later. Just start putting thoughts together for the baton pass in the far corner.

Be honest. Bleed all over the page. Don't edit, let it flow. Forget how much you hated writing in high school when a grade depended on it. Your past performance with pen on paper doesn't matter, but this does. It will matter to others and if you get on with it, you will discover how much it matters to you, too. It doesn't take physical fitness as it can be done anywhere, anytime, by anybody.

*Journaling is often meant to be private and directed at those specific issues that stressed or hurt, but it can also be full of wonderings and new ideas you are processing. Other writing can be directed at an audience. Your whole life story can be amazing and help others get in touch with your formative moments. Some have written a chronology of their most important choices and their consequences; how they have dealt with temptations; how they have been fooled by temptations hidden in their culture.*

Dallas Willard emphasizes the power we have to make choices and how critical they are in determining outcomes of our lives.[4] Describing the choices you have made or not made can benefit your kids in many ways as they have lived through many of the consequences. Just knowing that you had tough choices to make can normalize their own trials. Telling them how you would do it again given a second chance can guide them in their own tough choices with a long-range view of possible outcomes.

# Day 3

# A Windrunner's Journal

*I invite you to reread every sentence above which is **bold** and in **italics**. Write it down, in your own words if you wish, to remember it, reflect on it, discuss it, or even memorize it.*

## Avoiding Deathbed Regrets

Bonnie Ware, an author who spent many years working in palliative care, compiled a list of the five most common regrets expressed by the people she attended: I wish I'd had the courage to live a life true to myself, not the life others expected of me; I wish I hadn't worked so hard; I wish I'd had the courage to express my feelings; I wish I had stayed in touch with my friends; I wish I had let myself be happier. [5]

We can identify with many of those and try to take corrective action, but first notice how the source of most regrets is fear:

Courage to live life true to myself = fear of not being adequate or accepted

Hadn't worked so hard = fear of failure or inadequacy

Courage to express my feelings = fear of conflict or rejection.

Fear is the common denominator.

Some have told me on their deathbed: "I wish I hadn't taken life so seriously—worked so hard, but didn't really live—didn't play enough, laugh enough, and hug enough." The most frequent regret was, "I wish I had quit treatment sooner. The last few rounds of treatment weren't worth it. I have this nagging feeling they were a waste of precious time." Sounds like the Dragon used fear again and the illusion of a miraculous medical rescue to steal someone's life away.

Laughter and play releases endorphins just like a good workout. They are natural mood elevators and pain relievers, non-toxic and cheap. If you can't find anything to laugh about you are definitely taking life too seriously and you may as well be dead already. The slimy green assassin has taken your life and you don't even know it.

Remember the carefree life of childhood? Remember the creativity, the games and the laughter that were only possible because you hadn't learned how to fear yet? You didn't need to because you were still secure. To avoid regrets, you must learn to transcend the whole menagerie of your fears and you must do it now while there is still time left. You can deny that you have any and many people do, but being human they are invariably wrong.

There is one way to abolish fear and now is the time to do it. Then in many ways you can get back to being a kid again. That is to get to know Jesus and let Him guide your steps. There is security in knowing your purpose and your destiny and in trusting Jesus to guide you into both – a security that leaves no room for fear and at peace.

*Now is the time to know Him so well that you can trust him to show you the way. It is time for the next leg of your spiritual journey and to consider things of God. Let His words give free range to your imagination. Let the scars of the past leech out of you and feel your seasons change. The carefree wants to settle in. Childhood wonder wants to return. A new world awaits.*

# Day 4

# A Windrunner's Journal

*I invite you to reread every sentence above which is **bold** and in **italics**. Write it down, in your own words if you wish, to remember it, reflect on it, discuss it, or even memorize it.*

_____

_____

_____

_____

_____

_____

_____

_____

_____

_____

_____

_____

_____

_____

## WHY A SPIRITUAL JOURNEY NOW?

> *"There are two important days in your life: the day*
> *you were born and the day you figure out why."*
> — Einstein

Upon leaving the secure homes of our youth, we all became exiles in an uncertain and unsafe world. While a search for gratification and happiness commonly distracts, most people ultimately focus on recreating the security we once knew and still long for. We do it by investing ourselves in building relationships, assets and houses. Whatever success we achieve is quickly exposed as insufficient when disease comes on stage and demands a change in course. Disillusioned, but not defeated, many begin a pilgrimage for a spiritual homeland and discover an unexpected vitality on the journey long before they arrive.

Journeyers do come alive. They embrace that eager condition of "not knowing" and become curious. *Just living into that fundamentally anxious state of uncertainty is exactly what a 2007 study by Todd Kashdan and Colorado State psychologist Michael Steger found was a dominant characteristic of the happiest and most vital people.*[6] Try it. Embrace it. If you don't, soul-rot awaits. Your choice.

Happiness is not just about doing the things you like which are not always an option, but also about adventuring beyond your comfort zone. That is exactly what a spiritual journey is at the outset, an uncomfortable adventure, an invigorating tension. None of us completely arrive, but unlike most journeys, strength rises and pace quickens the further we go.

"It isn't reality that shapes your life but your view of reality."[7] *Ninety percent of your happiness is predicted not by your external world, but by the way your brain processes your reality.* God's story has a positive ending. Those who know it have a positive view of reality that shapes their lives even when they have cancer. That is worth investigating.

## REMEDIAL COURSEWORK

Recall the story I told in *Cancer's Bell Lap & The Dragon Behind the Door* about witnessing an extraordinary skier dancing on skis down the fall line between trees and over moguls when his heart stopped, and he turned into a ragdoll tumbling to a stop, motionless in death. I told you my first thought was that it seemed pretty cool to be skiing one moment in deep powder and only a heartbeat away from waking up in Heaven. Then I began to wonder if I would I really wake up and if I did, would I really be in Heaven? Would I really be ready to leave here or to arrive there? Would I have learned all that I needed to learn before leaving and would I have fulfilled all the responsibilities and opportunities of my life? Then it occurred to me that events like I had just witnessed cannot occur without God allowing them and not intervening to prevent them, but the being ready part would still been up to me.

*In Scripture, Jesus didn't cure every disease or prevent every calamity every time and He doesn't do so today. Who, when, and how He will bless us does not have to do with good works or the lack thereof. It isn't based on who has sinned or who hasn't, and it is not universal for those who claim His name, not at least in a form they always recognize. There is some divine calculus by which of His decisions are made that will always be a mystery to us, an equation which produces both individual and collective goodness, but is sometimes beyond the scope of our understanding or outside our timeframe.*

What if He sees catastrophic events unfolding before me and notes that there are a few more things He has planned for me to learn, a few more lives I need to interact with, a few more relationships with people He loves that I need to make right? He might just intervene to keep me around longer to get it right, not because I deserve rescue, but because I can be part of something good for someone else. If I'm not figuring it out or even motivated to figure it out, will He let that bell toll to get my attention—maybe even the cancer bell? I wonder?

I'm not suggesting He plans or creates cancer or any other awful hardship to wake us up, but when they happen He doesn't hesitate to use them for His own purposes. I know I have been pretty dense and slow in figuring some stuff out, enough so that He let the grizzly bear get in my face. It was kind of a "hit me over the head with a 2x4" moment. "WAKE UP NOW! I have something I'm trying to tell you!" He has also let some friends experience some pretty awful events that seemed to wake them up also.

Sometimes it seems the cancer has been ordained or permitted not for the benefit of a particular individual, but for the benefit of those whose lives that individual impacts. For example, a parent (of any age) can be profoundly impacted by cancer in the life of his child (of any age), or a spouse by their spouse, or a friend by their friend.

I don't pretend to know how God works in this arena, nor that any divine mathematics contribute to these stories. I know that I don't want any more 2x4 events in my life and I do want to learn from the echo of the bell ringing in the lives of my friends and patients. I want to let my soul grow by living as if I am dying. So, I'm starting to run my Bell Lap now and hope that I get far enough along so that if my biology fails me while climbing some mountain above the clouds or skiing the fall line in fresh powder or just nestled in the arms of the one I love, the Lord will just take me home rather than sending me back for some remedial coursework.

God says He has a plan for our lives, but how can that be when so much of the time we are not ready for what is next: time for getting a job, time for a baby to come, time to repair a roof, change a diaper, get cancer! That doesn't seem like such a great plan. Yet He has planned it that way or permitted it within His plan. **His perfect time is often *our not ready* time. From His perspective it is the *right* time for what He has planned.**

It didn't seem like the right time to Joseph when Mary learned that she was pregnant with Jesus or the right time for the guy who wanted to go bury his parents before following Jesus, or the right time for Jesus in Cana at the wedding when they ran out of wine, and I'm sure it does not feel like the right time to hear your bell ring or find yourself on your Bell Lap. But somehow *it is,* because God is letting it happen.

Strangely enough, you are now cast into an adventure you never planned, never wanted, and have no choice but to accept. It's a bit like your plane crashing in the jungle—no choice—gotta deal with it. Most folks will start praying. Good idea. ***The difference here is that if you know Jesus well, you can know for certain that the ending will be an amazingly good: either survival or heaven.*** Both sound great, but no one is eager to die to get to Heaven. However, the more you know about Heaven the more gentle the thought and then eagerness grows.

We can hold two divergent thoughts at the same time, both the expectation of survival in this life and a wondrous new life in heaven someday. Neither precludes the other and both preclude anxiety. How great is that.

## KEEP YOUR EYES OPEN

Your security up to this point may well have been based upon your plans for the future that you have been preparing for financially, physically, academically, and strategically. Now those plans are shot through with holes. Life as He designed it (perhaps better put as we free-will beings have responded to it) loves to catch us off guard. There must be a reason. I suspect it has something to do with teaching us something important, something we will ultimately be grateful for. Something He needs to take us out of our comfort zone, into the wilderness of the unknown to teach us where we are motivated to pay attention to our instructor i.e. Him.

**You can't hang on to your old plans and listen to God at the same time.** Enter the humanly unfathomable dynamic called surrender and give it all your plans, your dreams, all of you to Him. He may give a bunch of it back, but if He doesn't, it is only because He has something better in mind. That something may involve other people you don't even know yet. It is not likely you will see His plan at first, but give it time and keep your eyes open.

In the Jewish tradition the terminally ill are encouraged to put their affairs in order. There's something to be learned from these people with such a long recorded history of cohesive faith. In 2 Kings 20:1, the prophet Isaiah responds to ill King Hezekiah's inquiry, "This is what the Lord says: put your house in order, because you are going to die, you will never recover." Lucky Hezekiah, at least he got a warning. Will we?

No tradition counsels us when to put our affairs in order. To some it feels cowardly like giving up the fight and inviting death; hence they loath to do it. But where in any spiritual or medical tradition does it say that getting ready to die, hastens death? Nowhere! In reality, *those people who accept their inevitable death and are ready for it, are then free to run their Bell Lap as long and hard as they choose and to flight for life as long as they are able. They are empowered by knowing that they cannot lose and they are ready for either outcome!*

*When fear is gone and actually replaced with joyful anticipation of either outcome, all the biologic and psychic energy that was being consumed coping with the fear of death is salvaged and can be invested in both fighting for and actually living life!*

Fear begets fear. It creates delusions. When we are in its grasp, whether we recognize it or not, we are just as compromised as a paranoid schizophrenic. He actually hears and sometimes sees the voices in his head manipulating his thoughts and decisions, and threatening him with all kinds of horrid bodily harm. Our fears are just as real as his, but they speak more subtlety, maybe through friends, maybe through the profit motivated media. Each does it by somehow insinuating their messages into our consciousness and affecting our actions and decisions without our hardly hearing or recognizing them. Our Dragon is invisible.

*If one believes that accepting death at a visceral emotional level and not just at the flippant intellectual level will hasten death's arrival, then every thought of such acceptance will be deferred. Then the freedom of such acceptance is also deferred! Dragon wins. We lose.*

Deathbed confessions are common and are the purview of the rabbi, pastor or parish priest. Typically, they are delayed until nearly every spark of hope is extinguished. They are viewed by some as an important preparation for the transition from this world to the next, a means of repentance and final reconciliation with God. Hence, they are proffered as a source of comfort and completion, often with the unspoken expectation that it will pave the way to heaven. I'm not sure that works. It's a good start, but no guarantee.

A common form it might take is, "I acknowledge before You Lord, my God and God of my fathers, that both my healing and my death are in Your hands. May it be Your will to heal me in a complete recovery? If though I do die, may my death atone for my sins and transgressions that I have committed before You. Grant me a share in the world to come...."[8] In the Jewish rabbinic tradition, this will be followed by a series of deathbed testaments as with both the patriarch Isaac and his son Esau (Genesis 27) and Jacob with his twelve sons: the summons and subsequent blessings of the first son, the ethical instruction to the family, the ordering of material affairs, and transferring of pertinent responsibilities.

Today, often there is no script for the terminally ill, and they find themselves floundering in their dying just as much or more than their living. To the extent there is a script, it comes from the Hebrews and it is from these traditions that Christian and Western secular traditions have evolved.

The question is why wait until the final hour to deal with unfinished business, resolve lingering, long buried conflicts, bequeath blessings, proffer guidance, and shower and be showered with love, and then exit before the commemoration and celebration begins? Bummer! By that time, many are both sick and in the embrace of the unseen tentacles of uncertainty and anxiety orchestrated by fear that lurks in the shadows with the Dragon. Hardly the condition one would choose for giving one's best advice or celebrating one's whole life.

*Many who lead complex high pressure lives already are so accustomed to coping with and medicating their anxieties that they don't even recognize when that big brother ANXIETY, with his pal, FEAR have moved in. Others skillfully deny them both with a well-polished bravado. However, if these two are kicked out and gone, most will see them clearly for what they were, and they smile at the taste of a freedom they never knew existed. Those who smile run great Bell laps. There is no reason to wait for the Bell to start smiling and running. How does one get those monkeys, anxiety and fear off one's back? There is a better way than medicine to do that and we will talk about it. The question is, "Do you want to and when"?*

## WHY DEADLINES

*I believe in designing life, God has intentionally spliced clues into the fabric of every day to facilitate our understanding of His purposes. I suspect it is not an accident that the clues are hidden in plain sight in the metaphors of our existence and we are supposed to be looking for and considering these metaphors. If we do, they will shed light on many of life's mysteries. I got to wondering why God designed life with deadlines.* We all encounter them. In school and at work those deadlines prompt us to get something done and I suspect that is God's design for my life also. He wants me to get something done. Ever since the fifth grade when the deadline for my first term paper came I have been getting experience with the consequences of my proclivity for procrastination. That miserable experience became an ever overtaking wave of guilt that has propelled me forward ever since. Memories of the deadlines we have crashed into are like that.

# Day 5

# A Windrunner's Journal

*I invite you to reread every sentence above which is **bold** and in **italics**. Write it down, in your own words if you wish, to remember it, reflect on it, discuss it, or even memorize it.*

_____

_____

_____

_____

_____

_____

_____

_____

_____

_____

_____

_____

# Hearing the Bell Changes People

In January of 1989, Don Piper was driving fifty mph in his Ford escort across a narrow bridge across the Trinity River in rural Texas when he was struck head-on by an 18-wheeler.[9] The car and his body were crushed almost beyond recognition by grinding steel and flailing tires. When paramedics arrived, they found his mangled remains and detecting no pulse, pronounced him dead, and moved on to care for others.

While trained medics perceived Don absent from his body, he perceived himself in Heaven, only to be rudely and graciously returned to life ninety minutes later. Miraculously, he not only woke up, but he awakened to the song of a passerby who felt called to pray for a dead man.

Don offers his testimony to affirm that there is a heaven and that God is still in the business of doing miracles. More powerful than that is it changed his life in positive and extraordinary ways.

Researchers in the Netherlands studied 344 people with less dramatic, but none the less near-death experiences. They reported their findings in the Lancet, *The Journal of the British Medical Society*, December 2001. While skepticism can dismiss the commonalities of the survivors' experiences as the wishful thinking of oxygen starved brains, it seems profound to me how their lives subsequently changed. I can understand how a near death experience might well light a fire under them to accelerate their agenda in life, which for most would be an intensely self-centered pursuit of who they already were and what already mattered most to them. However, these near death survivors' whole personalities changed, and markedly: "they became more compassionate, giving, loving, and they lost their fear of death."[10]

Supercilious, innate biases can easily lead us to discount what people say, but it's harder to discount what actually happens in the lives of such a diverse group of people after a common experience—a brush with death and a glimpse of Heaven. Words alone can sound like the all-too-common scripted musings of what we wish for or may have been programmed to believe, but when lives actually change and in godly ways, one must sit up and pay attention.

It seems worthwhile to investigate this Heaven and this God before you have any near death experience of your own and while there is still time to make a change.

Invariably, someone asks, "Okay Doc, I get it that the spiritual stuff is really important, but is there anything I should be doing with my body and diet." The answer is, "Maybe, just don't let it be your primary focus. The Dragon will try to make it so. He can use it as one of the ploys in his denial delusion playbook. What I will tell you next can give you some worthwhile sense of control, but don't let the Dragon seduce you into thinking it is all powerful and distract you from what is more important."

# A Far Corner Reflection

If you have waited for the doctor to say, "We have nothing more we can do for you," you probably waited too long as an obedient supplicant of the medical menagerie. Whether you wait for the "no options decree" or you decide there are no options worth taking, when it happens it is at first a gut wrenching, chest tightening moment, but then something else happens. It is a release, a new freedom. One couple put it this way, "As what the doctor said sank in, I could feel something very heavy begin to lift. I felt as though we were free to live our life again. Bizarrely, life never felt so safe. Maybe I'm crazy, but I felt more freedom and not as though my life were being taken away. It was as though it was being given back to me. I was going to die but until then my life was completely my own."[11]

He discovered just the opposite of what he feared and expected. There was more room to live and to be fully alive. When the medical agenda diminished abdicating its primacy in dictating decisions, he could abandon man-made hopes and discover a kind of freedom he didn't even know was possible. He could live life exactly as he wished. In order to do that he had to learn to love the life he had exactly as it was and free from the burden of all the fantasies of what it might be. However, only a hope in heaven enables one to release hope on earth and experience such freedom.

# THE SIMPLICITY OF WINDRUNNER SPIRITUALITY

I am neither a theologian nor an expert at hermeneutics or a scholar of comparative religions. I am just a guy reminded that my death draws closer every day, especially as I meet others being brought down by cancer in their prime. I'm a guy who knows the opportunity to run the Bell Lap will come only once, and I want to start it now before I have to. To do so I recognize I need to accelerate my spiritual journey ASAP because I'm convinced, after watching Windrunners, that it is the only sure way to freely experience the *fullness of this life* every day until my last.

All I can relate to you is what I have learned from years of walking with Bell Lappers through the valley of the shadow of death with God or without Him. They have been heathens and hedonists, spiritualists, Christians, Buddhists, and New Agers. As I cared for them, I was not consciously comparing them or looking for anything in particular. Yet some patients distinguished themselves in such a way that I couldn't help but notice. My first response was amazement, my second was curiosity and my third was, "I want what they've got."

They had a peace and purpose I had never seen before. None brandished a philosophy nor claimed a group identity, but each treasured a relationship and a vision that had been built through trial and trepidation and had become intimate, trustworthy, and secure. Out of that relationship came vision and hope.

They were neither christianized nor churchified, but they were Christians. They went to a variety of different churches, but they worshipped one God. They described their journey as getting to know someone, not as becoming something. That someone was Jesus and the something was a Christian. Being known as a Christian didn't matter while knowing and trusting Christ was all that mattered. It was not enough for them to be in the right place, saying the right words, hands outstretched or on their knees. It was not enough until they were walking with Jesus twenty-four hours a day everywhere they went.

They spoke of Him not just as the codified and petrified historical Jesus whose words leap out off the pages of the New Testament, but as the very same Jesus who is also alive and well, at their side, guarding their hearts and guiding their lives.

One thing was for sure, theirs was no cliché religion. It wasn't about just going to church, saying all the right words, mouthing the prayers and petitions, clean living and tithing, though those are all good things, but also the ones that people can see, compare, and measure each other by.

It was about something going on in their hearts that only God can see and that was what made all the difference. It was about falling in love with Jesus. They recognized that it wasn't just standing in a pew singing hymns that pleases God, which it does, but rather an inward reality of holiness, contrition, commitment, and loving service that started with their families and spread outward from there.

When it comes to the Bell Lap, I call it passing the baton. It involves a shift in focus from what we want God to do for us to what God can do through us and discovering in that process He does his best work in us.

# Time to Write the Rest of Your Life's Script

Before you can bless others, you need to receive your own blessing. A good place to start would be to read Henry Nouwen's, *Life of the Beloved*. It is short, only 149 pages. You will be blessed. Get it now.

Here is your checklist from this chapter to really begin to write the rest of you life's script:

☐ Invite God to sift through all that is happening in your life and guide you to make peace with it.

☐ Let Him teach you how to forgive yourself as well as how to forgive those who let you down.

☐ Let Him support you in letting go and leaving behind the bits and pieces for which there is no explanation.

☐ Let Him heal your stuff and give you enough understanding and grace so that you can pass on a healthy baton.

☐ Remember the Lord doesn't collect or record the bad stuff; He forgives it and forgets it.

Your written thoughts need no beginning or end. Just start and they will lead you as the padlock comes off of your memories and secrets. You may be astounded at how thoughts and feelings that you didn't even know you had will come tumbling out and how, with the Lord's wisdom and grace, start making more sense.

Write about the people you have loved and why.

Write about the places you've lived and how they affected you.

Write about the things that made you laugh, cry and tremble.

Add your trials, your disappointments and your triumphs.

Permit yourself to be surprised as the details you have long forgotten start appearing on the page.

# CHAPTER 14

# THE WINDRUNNER BATON PASS

The question is why so many Christians live so poorly and insignificantly on the road to Heaven. There is often so little to admire much less imitate. Did they not know; did they not try or were they sidetracked?

Who are the true heroes? Those whose heroism isn't splashed in the headlines, but is printed in the lives it touches first hand. It doesn't hide its follies, but pursues adventures of goodness in spite of them.

For the heaven-bound Windrunners, there will be a grand reunion, but only after a sit-down talk with God at Heaven's Gate. He will ask: "How did you do with those children, spouses, and friends I entrusted to you?"

If there is anything you can do to mend or improve those relationships, you may as well do it now and start savoring the results and save yourself some embarrassment when you meet up with God. Completing those relationships will rest your heart and relieve theirs, both now and later. It will lessen the potential burden or sting of the things left unsaid both of which can conspire to haunt those left behind after your departing. Avoid complicating their grief. Remember that often the thing they will miss the most (or not) is the way you made them feel about themselves.

Howard Hendricks, long time professor at Dallas Theological Seminary, wrote, "Life is like a coin: you can spend it anyway you want, but you can only spend it once." He recounts something meaningful he learned during a decade as chaplain for the Dallas Cowboys. Mike Ditka, then Dan Reeves, Joe Gibbs, Tom Landry, and others had all said to him before a game, "Howe, I'm scared to death of this one. My team is going out to play *not to lose*." They told him, "Playing halfheartedly not to lose, instead of playing wholeheartedly to win, is the fastest way to defeat." In Christian life, halfhearted efforts instead of wholehearted obedience leads to defeat. He encourages us, **"There is no place in Christian life for retirement mentality. Just when our weary bones are seeking the rocking chair is when we ought to be most active for our Savior—running to win."**[1]

"As the Father has sent me, **I am sending you**. And with that he breathed on them and said 'Receive the Holy Spirit'" (John 20:21–22).

"His unique identity as Son of God was shown by the spirit when Jesus was raised from the dead, setting him apart as the Messiah, our master. Through him we received both the generous gift of his life **and the urgent task of passing it on to others**" (Romans 1:3–5 MSG emphasis added).

*You are not given the time you have left for your own sake; you have an evangelical mission to become a witness to hope.*

## How?

What is "it" and how do you pass it on? You do it best with a changed life. A cancer diagnosis can awaken one from the shallow complacencies in which we live, but unless the awakening leads to a changed life, there's not much of a baton to pass. Even when you discover that this life is not just about you, even when you become aware that you "are living in the middle of a story that was begun and will be continued by another-that being God,"[2] even when you willingly accept His commission to play your role in the story, most don't know how to pass their spiritual baton. It is not accomplished with words alone; they are not enough. They cannot take anyone further than you have already gone and can explain. The essential and most eloquent message is a changed life.

As God designed us and knew us long before it ever occurred to us to discover and know Him, it is He who will reveal the truth yet before us and how to pass it on. Jesus is committed to completing the story He has created for you and He does not intend for your part of the plot development to be lost. *God has revealed something about Himself in your story and He has written your life like a personal letter to your loved ones for whom it will bring special meaning.*

*You are the actor; He is the director. The message is His, the actions are yours. If you study the whole play and the trajectory of the plot, you will better be able to take His directions from the wings. If your life changes, it will make people curious, particularly with cancer in the equation. By the time you are coming down the home stretch, you will have their full attention. You will be in the spotlight on center stage. Make it count.*

By then there is no longer any neutral ground. Those days have passed. God is either in your life or He isn't. You have willingly surrendered your heart and soul to Him or not. You are letting Him guide and cheer you on or you are not? You are either letting Him inspire, educate, bless, rescue and heal or not. Those who are uninterested in what He offers and decline His involvement leave Him in a role He regrets and they cannot avoid that of judgment at Heaven's Gate.

# DAY 1

# A WINDRUNNER'S JOURNAL

*I invite you to reread every sentence above which is **bold** and in **italics**. Write it down, in your own words if you wish, to remember it, reflect on it, discuss it, or even memorize it.*

_____

_____

_____

_____

_____

_____

_____

_____

_____

_____

_____

_____

_____

## A Changed Life

A changed life means that part of Christ has become part of you. God wants to put that part of His glory on display. You can trust Him to show you how. When the going gets the toughest, the audience pays the most attention. *God's Spirit becomes more unmistakable in the weakness endured by an ailing and aging sage than in the strength and eloquence of those at the peak of their worldly game. It is more difficult to discern God's Spirit when it shares the stage with health and prosperity.*

It is easy when you are the one who is sick and dying and the doctors, nurses, family, and friends are all gathered around to feel that it is all about you, but it isn't. The run may be nearing its end, but it is not time to fade in the far corner. That is when so many races are won or lost. **Remember the relay runner doesn't get to stop running until the baton is securely past.** The Rolling Stones were wrong about "time"[3]—it's not on your side: get on with doing what you alone can do, run hard and pass your baton.

"God brings us to a place where He asks us to be our utmost for Him and we begin to debate. When we are young, health and wealth can distract us from the gravity of His request, so we question or ignore it. God's order has to work up to a crisis in our lives because we will not heed a gentler way."[4] **Give the kids the benefit of what you've learned through your crises and you will at least equip them with the foreknowledge to recognize their own providential crisis.**

## CHUCK – LIVING THE METAPHOR

I barely knew Chuck Austen, mostly through friends in Young Life, when I learned he was undergoing surgery. He had turned yellow with jaundice and the surgeons had found a cancer in the head of his pancreas. It was small and resectable, but subsequent examination in the pathology lab showed spread into adjacent lymph nodes. Bad news!

After the tumor obstructing his bile duct had been removed, he would recover and feel well for some time, but sadly undetectable seedlings, no larger than grains of sand, certainly remained and would grow to threaten his life. Sadder still, there was no known curative treatment, nor any treatment likely then to prolong his life.

I told him that even though past drugs had been poor for this disease, there were some new drugs and some research protocols that might be tried and maybe, just maybe, a cure could be found, but that would be a real long shot. Even though he was very fit and otherwise healthy, the treatment would be aggressive and would make him very sick.

*Then I told him about the Bell Lap. I told him on average our best estimate with or without traditional treatment was that he would have about nine months to live and he needed to decide how he wanted to invest the rest of his time, in treatment or in life. If he were to take treatment, he would sacrifice most of his feel-good time to side effects and yet very likely never achieve a cure. If on the other hand he were to spurn treatment, in all likelihood he would have several months of near-normal life then several of reasonable life and one month at the end of misery. To my surprise, Chuck grabbed on to the idea of running his Bell Lap toward life, rather than away from death.*

He was going to run his lap as best he could and not give up any of it to treatment toxicity. He knew what running was all about; he had done a lot of it playing football at the University of Oregon and later as a marathon runner. After leaving the hospital without chemotherapy in his veins, he went on to run another marathon with his daughter, maybe two.

Chuck also spent a lot of time with friends and family celebrating his life (and incidentally influencing others). He had committed his life to Jesus many years before and he knew where he was going. The peace that gave him was the wind at his back as he ran. He got his nine months and most of it was good; none was wasted. Coming down the home stretch, he gave each of his kids a leather baton, the very ones used in competition, each imprinted with encouraging words of fatherly wisdom and a scripture. Throughout that time the same peace and joyful anticipation radiated from his face as it had from Wendell's and Sally's.

# Day 2

# A Windrunner's Journal

*I invite you to reread every sentence above which is **bold** and in **italics**. Write it down, in your own words if you wish, to remember it, reflect on it, discuss it, or even memorize it.*

_____

_____

_____

_____

_____

_____

_____

_____

_____

_____

_____

_____

## CONNIE – FOR GOD'S PLEASURE

Twenty years later, Chuck's close friend and mine, Connie Jacobson developed the same symptoms with the same cancer. Secure in the arms of the same God, Connie made the same no treatment decision, but it wasn't an easy decision. It took some time to sort out and wrestle with God about it. He came within just a few hours of taking chemotherapy before the answer was clear not only to him, but independently to trusted prayer partners. He had pondered all the Bell Lap stuff, toxicity issues, and response rates with chemotherapy. Then he processed it all in community with close friends and family.

For his seventy years, he had led a vital life actively engaged with his kids, grandkids, community leaders, and hundreds of men in a ministry called Telious that he had started thirty-five years earlier. Connie was remarkably healthy despite his cancer, and **he could have tolerated even aggressive chemotherapy, but it would have cost him precious *time, energy,* and *focus*. Being a leader of men, a father, grandfather, and husband, he felt called to be the epic man's man, but in the end decided to be God's man!**

Fear of death did not drive his decision making, but he struggled with what kind of leader he wanted to be. At first, he signed up for chemotherapy in part because society expects men to be courageous and because courage is so often defined as fighting, with the greatest paradigm of courage being fighting for one's life in a theater of war. A battle with cancer is no less daunting and a parallel is often drawn. Many men clambering to the call of courage and others are pushed by those around them to the front lines of chemotherapy.

Connie knew that fighting for his own life would surely bring all kinds of accolade, but he chose to fight a different sort of battle- one with convention, and with societal expectations. *He came to recognize that just fighting cancer can steal away the very life you are fighting for. Sometimes there is not enough life left to waste on a fight—even a good one.*

After having signed up for the chemotherapy to the applause of his wife and children, he wrestled prayerfully with that decision throughout the night before the planned treatment was due to start. On waking, the angst was gone and that peace that he experienced so many other times after a long talk with Jesus had returned and he knew chemotherapy was not the right choice for him. When his wife's eyes opened and before he could speak, Judy told him that the Lord had changed her mind also. Then they got a call from their daughter Lori to say that during the night Jesus had changed her mind as well. With that, another Windrunner came powering out of the near corner and down the backstretch.

Do you remember the pivotal scene in *Chariots of Fire,* the movie made about the life of Eric Liddell, a devout Scottish Christian and track star, respected for both his speed and his convictions at the 1924 Paris Olympics? (If you don't, find it now, you must see it. You need this visual image and the music – and you will love the movie.) Eric is rounding the far corner of the 400 meter race, the home stretch is before him, he throws his head back, lengthens his stride, the theme music crescendos, and a joyful smile breaks across his face. We hear and see what Eric felt while sprinting toward the finish line, **"When I run, I feel God's pleasure."**

*That was Connie on his Bell Lap every day after he loosed his grip on the world's final agenda and grabbed even harder onto God's.* The Lord filled his days with purpose: family gatherings and words for every child and grandchild, meetings with young men, old men, community leaders, clergy, and friends— always with a message which I will paraphrase. "God has had a plan for my life all along and this is part of it. Despite hardships, sometimes pain, sometimes tears, God has always been with me and He is with me now, and it is all good. I'm looking forward to seeing Him face-to-face."

You could see the light of Jesus and the hope of heaven in his eyes every day, an indelible validation of Connie's words to all of us over many years. When the war for your soul is won and you know it, you don't need to be distracted by battles with cancer where only your body is at stake. The Dragon can yell discouragement, defeat, and things to fear, yet it all falls on deaf ears. Connie could have chosen to waste his time and energy fighting a battle he could not win against metastatic pancreatic cancer, but instead he chose to give his all running a race coached by

Christ that he could not lose. I will not soon forget his example and hope that I may someday run as well.

There is something terribly significant going on here. Jesus repeatedly tells us He wants to be first in our lives. He wants our allegiance to Him to be above all else: worldly achievements, family, our own safety, and even our lives. He tested Abraham with specter of sacrificing his precious son, Isaac. He tested Jesus with the specter of death on a cross. He lets our own mortality test each of us. He is watching what is going on in our hearts as death draws near just as He watched Abraham as he walked toward the Mount of Moriah with a bundle of sticks, a knife, and Isaac. Just as He watched His own Son, Jesus anguish in the Garden of Gethsemane.

Abraham's response to God was, "I'm listening." Jesus' was, "Not My will but Yours." The terrible prospects before them did not alter their attentiveness or their obedience nor did it for Connie, Chuck or Wendell. For their willing hearts and obedient feet, they all were blessed.

*No one can predict what God will say to you at that crucial time, but it seems prudent to be listening carefully and be willing to sacrifice what is most precious, your life, to respond to His call.*

# DAY 3

# A WINDRUNNER'S JOURNAL

*I invite you to reread every sentence above which is **bold** and in **italics**. Write it down, in your own words if you wish, to remember it, reflect on it, discuss it, or even memorize it.*

_____

_____

_____

_____

_____

_____

_____

_____

_____

_____

_____

_____

_____

# IT'S NOT JUST ABOUT STOPPING/ FOREGOING TREATMENT

Some of my examples are about people who decided to stop or never take cancer therapy. One should not conclude that I am proposing that it is universally unwise or even unchristian to take aggressive anticancer treatment. Not at all. Many took such chemo and usually did better than statistics would predict, but only when God gave them a leading and the peace to do so. My point is quite different. I am saying ask for leadership and listen.

*It is not the decision to decline or discontinue therapy that makes a Windrunner, but it is the peace and knowing that enables the decision and the purpose behind it that does. This purpose is never about giving up; it is about the ultimate giving over. It doesn't take courage because the fearful uncertainty is gone, the Dragon's fire breath has been extinguished. The Dragon is still alive, but irrelevant. For the Windrunners, a new life has already begun.*

After such a decision, it becomes easier to distinguish the true Windrunners from everyone else. Until that decision some folks can fake peace pretty well, even fool themselves, but afterwards, when delicious peace has settled in, there is no need to fake it.

There are many Windrunners who appropriately choose aggressive therapies up front that have achieved remission or cure, but I have never seen one do it as a last ditch effort. **Nor have I ever seen God swoop in with a last minute deathbed**

**miracle to save someone holding out for it. Let that idea go and focus your attention on Heaven.** If God plans to rescue you on death's doorstep, He will do it anyway. He won't back off because you are looking forward to being with Him in Heaven instead of trembling in the "name-it-and-claim-it" angst waiting for your own requisite miracle.

It is difficult for an outsider to distinguish such Windrunners from anyone else who is happily in remission or cured because everyone looks and feels pretty much the same in happy-snappy land. The Dragon is still present assuring they have some PTSD or PTCD (post traumatic cancer distress) that they cannot escape. Even though the Windrunners actually experience less angst and more peace, more direction and certainty in their lives, the peace they feel is often not as discernible from the outside until they come face-to-face with their own death or some other terrible trauma. However they feel it every day on the inside.

## LISA – KINGDOM OUT-WORKINGS

Lisa tells me she couldn't make it without the Lord, but it is still hard sometimes. Before cancer rang her own bell, she had been getting in Bell Lap shape running alongside husband Dave on his. She sent me a quotation that the Lord seemed to have brought to her which defined her experience. "When God comes to you wrapped and wreathed in clouds, and in storms, why should we not recognize Him, and say, 'I know You, God;

and I will not flee You; though You slay me, I will trust in Thee?' If a man could see God in his troubles and take sorrow to be the sweet discipline of a bitter medicine that brings health, though the taste is not agreeable, and if one could so look upon God, how sorrows would make him strong! (Henry Beecher)."

She went on saying, "This resonates with me because from the very beginning I believe that Dave would not have cancer without God's permission and that His permission is not capricious, but has a purpose. I wish I understood that purpose better than I do; I can only pray for more understanding and trust in Him. I have come to more fully appreciate that God is really not about my fulfillment or happiness or whatever, He is about His kingdom purposes in this world. Sometimes that means that things happen in the course of the outworking of His plan that make no sense to me, and are even painful. But He is the Potter and I am the Clay—He can make me what He will. As if He needed my permission!"

## ANOTHER REASON

There is another reason why passing the *"what-you-know-about-God baton"* is so important and why you must spend much of the backstretch preparing to do it and it's all about you. It is exciting to think that what you will invest in the next generation will grow with compounding interest into every generation beyond, but it is equally exciting to anticipate what the preparation will do in you. It compels you discover what you really know and believe, how you got there, and then to put the pieces together in a way that others can grasp.

Every attempted explanation will reveal gaps in your understanding which will compel you to figure them out and your faith will grow in the process. It really matters just as much for you as it does for them. God will pick up with you in Heaven where He leaves off with you in life so none of today's struggles to understand are wasted.

God calls us to hold our light high and let it shine. It is His light, you don't need to create it, but you darn well better not hide it or be ashamed of it. Jesus didn't mince words on how He feels about that, "If anyone is ashamed of me and my words in this adulterous and sinful generation, the Son of Man will be ashamed of him when he comes into his Father's glory with the holy angels" (Mark 8:38).

*Even if your spiritual journey has not taken you as far as you wish, or as far as it seems to have taken others, pass it on, even with all its uncertainties and doubts. Whatever seedlings of faith you have found, plant them in the soil of another's soul. God will nourish them there and perhaps they will burst into full flower in their generation. Only a few can bestow much worldly wealth upon their children and that, as often as not, defeats their kids' ambition or retards their spiritual growth. Transmitting even the beginning of your spiritual journey is worth more in eternal terms than that.*

# DAY 4

# A WINDRUNNER'S JOURNAL

*I invite you to reread every sentence above which is **bold** and in **italics.** Write it down, in your own words if you wish, to remember it, reflect on it, discuss it, or even memorize it.*

_____

_____

_____

_____

_____

_____

_____

_____

_____

_____

_____

_____

_____

## EXPERIENCE/EXCUSES

Inexperience and disability are not an excuse if God is calling you to something even if it seems outlandish or beyond your ability. Walk into it as best you can and let God show you what He has in mind. His strength and creativity can amaze you provided you take it a day at a time and don't get hung up on your own preconceptions of what He is doing.

*When God sets your life on a new course, it is easy to look out in that direction and conclude He is heading for some destination/goal you can see like a distant mountaintop straight ahead. It is so easy to jump to such a conclusion and in effect say, "God, okay, I've got it from here," and bolt toward the mountain you see only to encounter all kinds of strife along the way and to then discover when you get there that God is not there. Had you listened for guidance day by day you would have discovered something quite different. God's plan was actually to go in the direction of the mountain then veer left through a hidden valley toward another mountain that you cannot as yet see. Don't limit God to only those solutions you can see or imagine or you will risk getting out in front of Him and missing out on something only He can think up.*

## Beyond Words

"To hear is to forget, to see is to remember," opined Nathan Mukuka, a thirteen-year-old Zambian, talking about the impact on him of seeing a godly mentor die in peace.

> *Moses said to the Lord, "Oh Lord, I have never been eloquent ... I'm slow of speech and tongue." The Lord said to him "who gave man his mouth ... Is it not I, the Lord? Now go; I will help you speak and will teach you what to say." Then the Lords anger burned against Moses and he said,' what about your brother Aaron? You shall speak to him and put words in his mouth; I will help both of you speak and will teach you what to do."* (Exodus 3:10-14)

That is exactly what God is saying to each of us, just be prepared to do your best. Even if you're not sure, give it a try. The Lord hates a slacker. If you still feel inadequate like Moses, there must be another plan and you had best find it.

## Recruit

Connect your kids to those you admire and trust who can speak for you into their lives. Commission friends to do just that.

Go to them individually or call them altogether and ask them to shepherd your kids. Divide up the kids. Divide up the areas of influence. Divide up the decades. Then ask for volunteers and commitments. It is not an accident those people are in your life. God put them there for times like this.

## SHOW

*Words cannot convey the most important and enduring message that is written in the confident countenance of one dying peacefully in the Lord's arms.* It is a message time cannot erase nor the fears of death destroy. Visual images are recorded more indelibly in memory and with more eloquence, complexity and accuracy than words. Don't hide away during the end times. Call family to your side.

*Children won't need to fear life, if they see their parents don't fear death.* What you say matters, but what they see matters more. It's not just what you do, but it's what's in your eyes and on your face, those windows into your soul that matters the most. It's not something that you can fake. Swagger and bravado are not what I'm talking about; peace, purpose, and destiny are.

# LARRY – HEAVENLY EXPECTATIONS DOESN'T MEAN GIVING UP

It is harder when both spouses aren't in the same place at the same time. At the outset they seldom are. Sometimes the one with cancer lags behind their healthy spouse who is the Windrunner and sometimes it's the other way around. However, the love and peace of the Windrunners is so infectious that they often end up running together side-by-side.

Larry was a man's man, but one whose strength was quiet. He wore his grit with gentleness; it was a kind that didn't need to show off. He was in his fifties when he developed a peculiar pain radiating along the side of his neck to his ear and a dry cough that wouldn't go away.

As an insulin-dependent diabetic, he had become attuned to his body. He had to be to live the physically aggressive life that called to him: mountain biking and hiking in the summer and skinning up the backcountry on rondenee skis to find untracked powder in the winter. He loved the mountain solitude and he loved the companionship of his sweetheart and wife, Val. As a family, they ran a landscape supply business which sustained a life that was hard, but good until the cough and ear pain brought him to his physician and then to me.

His effervescent spirit greeted me when I first walked in the room. Soon we discovered that the pain was radiating from a large lymphomatous mass, hidden in the middle of his chest. To my surprise, his spirits didn't change when I told him about it. I was blown away just like with Wendell. I knew that either something special was going on with this guy or he was just out of touch with reality.

I guess you could say he was both. As I came to learn, he lived in another reality. I suppose you could call it, "God's dimension." He participated in life as if an actor in a play: someone else was writing the script and crafting the plot. He knew that as good as the drama of his life was with Val and their sons, it was only part of something much bigger that would play out in eternity.

At the beginning, Val wasn't in quite the same place. Larry said, "She cocked her head one way then the other with a worried, even dismayed look on her face, looking at me like I had a carrot stick out my ear or something askew asking, 'Why are you so happy? Why aren't you depressed?'"

Larry and Val undertook a heroic fight against the cancer which included aggressive chemotherapy, chest surgery, and radiation all appropriately aimed at cure. The battle produced a complete remission, but it only lasted a year when the Bell tolled again, but much louder and there was no mistaking it. Plausible deniability, cloaked in the hope of cure, was gone. We had given it our best and recognized that ***backup therapies seldom cure cancer any more often than second string quarterbacks win games.***

Larry had lived life as a lover. He brought light and affection into everyone's life, and he was loved back. I doubted he had much repenting or forgiving to do, or many relationships to heal, but he said he had some. He confessed that his self-sufficiency and self-reliance had left some things he needed to surrender and some apologies he needed to make. His macho had hidden some things in his heart that he needed to share and he still had some fathering of grownup sons left to do. They had worked with him in the business and he felt that he needed to figure out how to become more of a mentor than a boss and he knew he didn't have much time left. He knew the backstretch was behind him and he was into the far corner, so he was going to get after it.

Meanwhile, he wasn't going to let the cancer steal a single day of gusto from his life. Many days he would get out for one of his favorite thirty-mile rides through Orting and when the snow fell light and fresh and deep he would respond to the mountains call. Even with the growing lymphoma in his chest strangling his wind at 7000 feet, his gusto never lessened as he beckoned me down one of his favorite runs, Right Angle Ridge at Crystal Mountain. Sucking air, but grinning broadly he panted out, "I'll bet the powder is this good in heaven—maybe even better."

**Even when a doctor tells you that the end will come, most folks still feel pretty good in the far corner, and it is hard to believe the truth enough to act on it.** Larry did, and because he made his decision early and spurned taking last-ditch chemo-therapy which seldom works, he had enough time to do it well. He downsized his life by selling their large home and thereby salvaged precious time and energy that would have otherwise been spent dealing with its complexities. There are not many things someone with cancer can do themselves to create more of those precious commodities of time and energy, but that is one. Others who have acted similarly have been amazed to discover how much energy they had been expending just buying and maintaining their stuff and what freedom arrived when they quit.

For Larry it took stepping over the ego so typical of men that clings to more, bigger, and better in order to do something loving for his wife. When he did, it got her positioned securely for the time when she would be on her own and it freed up time, stamina, and resources they were able to invest in more precious pursuits. Next, he passed the reins of his business to his sons and stopped being their boss, to become an advisor and counselor.

*He was passing the baton and bringing a chapter of his life to a successful close, writing it with his own hand as is only possible when you start early enough to ensure you can get it done. Maybe, just maybe the Lord gave him some extra time because he was doing such a good job and following God-given directions. None of those decisions were easy. I listened to him struggle with them as they took him to his knees. Then he got up, not only knowing what to do, but wanting to do it. Peace and purpose had arrived. How sweet it was.*

# IN THE BLINK OF AN EYE

In *BLINK*[5], Malcolm Gladwell informs us that we have two kinds of attitudes: conscious attitudes which are those things we choose to believe, and unconscious attitudes which are those things that immediately tumble out before we have a chance to think – ones we may not actually be aware of. Unconscious learning is going on all the time, some of it is good and some not so good. Sometimes you can know more in the blink of an eye than after months of study through a process scientists call "rapid cognition."

The way we usually learn is to make observations, formulate hypotheses, test them, make more observations, and then add it all up to reach conclusions. Sometimes that happens rapidly and unconsciously and enables an appropriate response even though we don't know why or where it came from. Gladwell tells us it is called our "adaptive unconscious" which quickly processes all kinds of visual and auditory information. It helps people reach conclusions even before they know it—even before they've been able to consciously sort it all out. That is the way it is with "the peace of God that surpasses all understanding" (Philippians 4:7). You know it when you see it, but you can't explain it or describe it with words. It's a God thing.

I recognized it when I cared for certain people like Larry, but I didn't know what it was, where it came from or how they got it. That was before I had ever read Philippians 4:7. Now I can sense it soon after meeting someone and I know what it is. They are at peace with who they are and with letting you be who you are. They are at peace with what life has in store. They are at peace with not knowing what life will do next, but confident that God will be in it and it will be good.

## TOUCH

There are times when words are inadequate to explain what we feel or want to say. We need to rely upon the rapid cognition and adaptive unconscious of those we teach. We need to *show* rather than to speak in order to teach a golf swing, tennis serve, or how to live a life in peace. That is why Christ said "follow Me" not just believe what I say. Actions, tone of voice, and body language all speak a truth that words can only imitate. Even beyond showing comes *touching*.

Something happened over 100 years ago to many families that came across the Atlantic and seems to be happening more with succeeding generations. We are losing touch with touch. Why it has happened doesn't matter, but the consequences do. Those who have lost touch as part of their relational vocabulary with family and friends are crippled when a life is in peril. Touches, squeezes, hugs, and kisses all speak volumes beyond words. Regain them.

***Touch needs no time for analysis or interpretation by the literal brain, but connects directly to the heart. Without it,***

*you have to figure out what to say and how to say it so it won't be misinterpreted. Then you must stumble and choke out the words, then wait while the recipient dealing with medicated or metabolic brain fog tries to sort out whether the message they received was the message you sent. Touch bypasses it all.*

Often I have watched families standing or sitting across the room from their bed ridden loved one. It's hard to talk about much else than the weather when you're 8 to 10 feet apart, which of course is a safe distance for all those who can't quite find the words they would like to say. Often nothing gets said.

I encourage both parties to get closer, on the bed, in it or beside it and get a hold of each other. Touch is like a hard drive downloading. It sets a context of intimacy and requires no words. It can bridge the years, step over bitterness, and knock aside the discord that divides. Sometimes it says, "I love you," sometimes, "I forgive you," and sometimes, "just draw closer, come to me, I have so much to tell you." It is part of the vocabulary of intimacy for which there's no parallel. Bring it back.

It is already the most eloquent and natural communication of many, but is available to all. It is easy for women and it's easy for real men. It's hard for men who are insecure about their manhood, but then so is everything else. Start reaching, touching, hugging, and kissing soon - and practice often.

# "One Living Sermon Is Worth 100 Explanations"[6]

Who you are throughout the Bell Lap, with the baton pumping, the fatigue showing, and the symptoms growing, will be picked up unintentionally by all those around you. A message about the most feared and misunderstood subject in life, dying, will be stored indelibly at a subconscious level and can influence thoughts and behaviors of others far in the future. A receptive heart will receive your message on the first pass, but for others it will take time and repeated exposure. For some it will be easily missed or overridden by crushing emotions. So don't save what you have to show or tell until the very end.

## Expectations

What do college kids do when they are looking forward to moving to a new city for college? They talk about it. What do we all do before going on a far-off vacation? We talk about it to all our friends. We talk about everything we've heard and imagine with an enthusiasm that becomes infectious. The listeners go away with, "Gee, I wish I was going, too" attitude and a wistful, "I hope I get to go someday."

Heaven is a whole lot cooler than college away from home or any far-off vacation. It is something to be excited about and something to tell others about. If they are like most people I know, they don't know much about it and have probably never given it much thought. Yet they're destined to have innumerable precarious experiences that would be ever so much more tolerable if they knew that even if the worst of their imaginings comes true, they would just be heaven bound. "A teaspoon of sugar helps the medicine go down," sang Mary Poppins. Heaven is real and it is really worth look forward to. There are people who will never really know that unless you tell them.

Read the chapter on Heaven, mull it over, and read it again. Pray for understanding. Then read it again. Let God's promises settle into your soul. Let hope germinate and grow. When you do, tell your loved ones about it and how you are already looking forward to the reunion you will all have there.

The world becomes impatient with grief and if that is all you leave your family with, they are destined to have some lonely dark days ahead in their impatient world. There is so much you can do to limit the grief they will experience. Start sharing your illness as soon as you can with them and process all the feelings and fears it creates with them. It may take all of the backstretch to figure yourself out, and to get going on your journey with Jesus just to arrive in the place of promise and hope. If you get on with it, then by the time you're rounding the far corner you will be ready to share with them your hopes in Heaven and God's promises. By then, if you have given them enough time to process everything along with you, they too will be ready, able, and probably eager to learn of your hope. When they see your confidence, it may inspire them on their own spiritual journey. Then **hope can overtake sadness before it turns irretrievably into grief.** They will need that hope to turn a despondent goodbye into *hasta la vista* or "until I see you again." As one of the departing put it, "I'll have the burgers on the barbeque ready and waiting."

## GIVING AND SERVING

Many of us have our lives structured around getting more money, more stuff, more security, more health, more love, and ultimately more control for our families and ourselves. We seldom think about it that way because it sounds too self-centered. So we disguise it all with various virtuous names, but just the same, living without them leaves us out of control and forever anxious.

When "getting" shifts to "giving" that all goes away. Giving is totally in your control! Givers are not anxious, fearful, or desperate. Actually they are happy, partly because it is so much fun to see the happiness their gift creates and partly because it feels so good to be so powerful. Not powerful to manipulate, but full of the power to decide where and how to give yourself away.

**We know that in natural disasters, those who get involved like doctors and nurses, caregivers and cooks, those who find a job to do and take on responsibilities have a better chance of survival.** It was seen in the Nazi death camps where privation and cruelty affected them all equally. Those who helped and served survived longer!

My wife, Suzanne, sees it in her counseling practice. Those withering from personal trauma or tragedy often experience a transformational healing of body and spirit when they get outside themselves to focus on others.

Illness limits physical resources or stamina to do many things, but you can use your words. They take no more energy then you are already using just to breath and can make an extraordinary difference in the lives of others. If you are impressed watching what God is doing in your life and the lives of those around you, stop spectating. God didn't create you to be a bench warmer. Get off it and into the game.

*You may not think you have the gift, but that is only because you haven't found your natural niche. Go find it. No one hits a home run the first time at bat. Swing away and with God's grace you will start connecting. Every day you have an opportunity to affect a life, and someday what you say may help save one. Don't wait. Get involved. Small things matter. They add up to big things. That is what passing the baton in the far corner is all about.*

Finding one's niche involves finding one's purpose. The cancer is part of a bigger picture and did not take place in a void. If one survives into remission, for however long it lasts, it is because there is still a purpose to it all—purpose that will fuel the words and service to others. We don't need to know the why;

we only need to trust that we do not suffer in a void and that God will use our experience for His ultimate glory.

We are hardwired for sacrificial giving and for protection of our offspring. We are also hardwired for survival and that usually means to be getters. Therefore, giving and serving others beyond family is a learned behavior. If you are on the Bell Lap, it is the last chance under your control to go beyond yourself and ask God how He wants you to serve and give yourself away. It requires a willingness to let Him change your heart. If you do, a distraction with death can turn into a new passion with a purpose. Curiously its byproduct is happiness. Imagine that even though you are the one dying! Lon could and did.

## LON – RUN ALL THE WAY

Lon Woodard was another who came into the far corner choosing to serve, not to prove anything nor to seek approval nor earn his way into heaven, but because he had experienced God's grace and already knew he was loved and accepted. I didn't know him well, but I got to be one of his coaches on the backstretch.

Lon was not a man of the cloth; he was a man of the gridiron. He had played for Don Coryell on the legendary San Diego State team and then for the Saints. He was a giant of a man, but a gentle spirit. One didn't need to be around him long to figure out that he had no short supply of courage. He was savvy and daring in business having made and lost a fortune and made another. He was a backwoods fly-fishing guide and a friend to many.

Somewhere along the line he had met Jesus and joined a group of guys in Ketchum to share life and study the Bible on Thursday mornings where his candor and humility built the kind of bonds men cherish, but seldom speak about. When he got colon cancer, he decided he would take chemotherapy if it would give him some extra quality time and it did. When he relapsed in the far corner, he looked shrewdly at the statistics and thought about what he wanted his Bell Lap to look like. He decided the chance of benefit wasn't worth what it would cost him in hassle and side effects.

I'm not sure *he* had big plans for the rest of his life, but he suspected that God might. Lon didn't want to waste any time on side effects or sidelined in the hospital. He didn't want pity he wanted significance, so he gave every last drop his energy to God. He opened his calendar and God created plans for him all about serving his family and community.

Enduring fatigue with never a complaint, he abandoned humanity's love affair with comfort and he dedicated the last six months of his life to planning a men's fellowship retreat.

Like the apostle Paul who called his own life a daily death, Lon joined in the paradox, "Sorrowful, yet always rejoicing; poor, yet making many rich, having nothing yet possessing everything" (2 Corinthians 6:10). The Lord is my helper, I will not fear. Two days before he died, Lon was still sending e-mails to friends reminding them of retreat details that needed tending.

Windrunners never stop running just because they're tired or looking forward to the other side of the finish line. They don't need to complain or make excuses. That is what people expect. Instead, they get to surprise everyone in the stands with the quality of their effort and the One who supports it.

## BEWARE

If you find Jesus, and start running your Bell Lap with Him, people will notice and so will your enemy. If you're about to make a great baton pass, ole Redlegs will notice and he will act. If you don't believe he exists, you will never see his attack coming let alone know how to resist it.

Recognizing that the devil by every name, Satan, Beelzebub, Father of Lies, Great Dragon, Fallen Angel, Antichrist is real is even more mind blowing that believing God is real. The Scriptures are very clear on this. The devil stalks the earth (1 Peter 5:8). You may have lived through the consequences of his deceptions before. You may have even have triumphed over them, but he will take one last shot at you to prevent you from passing on what you know to the next generation. It may come as feelings of denial or of a worthlessness destiny in the glue factory, or timidity, fatigue or just that ever creeping procrastination. Watch out for it and with God's help overcome it.

*You may never have thought of yourself as one doing the devil's work, but if you are still harboring any bitterness or any deception, you are. If he ties the tongue in your mouth and your hands to your sides preventing you from loving, hugging, and giving, then he has stopped you at the line of scrimmage. You've fumbled and missed your only living chance to move the ball down the field for the next generation. You are not going to have much to say for yourself at Heaven's Gate.*

Shakespeare put it most eloquently, "Tis now the very witching time when churchyards yawn and hell itself breathes out contagion to this world." The contagion is not a virus or bacteria, but every bit as infectious and invisible, indeed more so. The contagion of hell is the fear of death which once inoculated in one life can spread like either the Ebola virus or the bubonic plague, from one life to another and consuming them all.

The devil's contagion does not die out with the death of its victim. It is transmitted generation to generation, to the unborn, and the yet to be conceived. Once conquered, that conquest creates an immunity which also can be passed on instead. If you become a conqueror, you have got to pass it on.

The cause of the bubonic plague or "Black death" was a mystery in the fifteenth century. Now we know that is caused by Yersinia Pestis, a bacterium passed in the saliva of rat fleas to humans. Only those who developed antibodies to the bacteria became immune and survived. Curiously, that immunity can be transferable from one person to another by a transfusion of serum. However, it is not enough for the one who is immune to donate their serum. The one who is ill needs to receive it. So offer what you have with gentleness like Christ did, never bombastically.

The baton is something you offer. The rest is up to God working in the heart of the next runner who gets to choose whether to grab it. Don't let the Dragon shame you into thinking it is all up to you and trick you into making a hard sell no one will buy.

Immunity to the fear of death seems entirely mysterious to anyone who doesn't have it. It comes only through the words of the one who has Himself conquered death, Jesus. Go to Him. Receive His words like a transfusion and let them fill you up. Perhaps it will take a series of inoculations, a series of trust experiments before you can trust all that He has to say. When you do, you will discover an immunity that will let you run freer, faster, longer, and more joyfully than you ever thought possible.

Beware though. Even if you defeat fear and rest in God's assurance of heaven, the enemy can sideline you in other ways. One of the most common is with the question "why." Unanswered, it doesn't send you to Hell, but it can distract you so that you neither live joyfully nor pass the baton.

## DAVE – HURDLING THE UNKNOWABLE

Dave is one of the living Windrunners, but there were hurdles on the track right off the starting line. Not until he cleared them could he lengthen his stride and run like the wind. He told me about the one that brought him to a standstill.

The diagnosis of his high grade prostate cancer was devastating and confusing to him largely because he couldn't understand **why** it had happened. He had walked with God most of his life and been vigilant about his health, avid in exercising, cautious in eating, and had followed both his physician's and naturopath's advice. Cancer didn't make sense biologically or spiritually.

He told me he couldn't move on with his life or his God until he abandoned the quest for why. *He couldn't feel free until he realized that not only would he never know why, but that he is not meant to know why. More importantly he doesn't really need to know why in order to craft his life going forward. There is meaning and purpose in what has happened, but it is not hidden in the WHY IT HAPPENED, but rather in the WHAT HE WOULD DO WITH IT!*

He chose to keep making his life count by serving others, not by building a monument to himself, but by building one to God with his life. He is still doing just that and it is fun to watch. I have learned from his experience and been blessed firsthand by his efforts. I have been on the track with him running by his side, skiing powder, climbing mountains, and chasing elk. While I have no reason to believe he will reach the finish line before me, he is running stronger. Confronting cancer does that!

## GALE – GRACE INFUSED LIVING

Gale and David were my mentors and I was their doctor. I knew medicine and they knew Jesus, so we took turns listening. One day, I asked Gale to share with me something they had learned from her cancer experience. She responded, *"Our gracious and loving heavenly Father has freed us from that delusion that we have control over making long-term plans. I now know that when we make them, I must hold onto them lightly and not get too attached to them so that I won't become unraveled if they don't work out. I wish I had learned this earlier life. This is a strange stretch of road we are on and we do not know which way it will bend, but we know where it ends up! That makes all the difference."*

I told you earlier about our friend Gale who had worked as a Young Life Beyond Malibu mountain guide, who sang in our wedding, worked in our cancer center and moved to Lebanon with her new husband David to bring the words of Jesus to a hurting Moslem world. There she got a vicious skin cancer which aggressive surgery and chemotherapy could not control.

If faithfulness and good works were criteria for divine physical healing, this angel of a woman would certainly be with us still, but she is not. While never cured, she was ever blessed. She survived and lived an exceptional life for years longer than any of her doctors ever expected.

Gale said she couldn't avoid wondering whether she would receive divine healing and she could easily find scripture to stand on which seemed to promise that she would. She always cautioned herself about doing that. **"I've got to beware of using Scripture as a blank check for my own needs."**

Unfortunately, I have seen others trip up doing that. When they do, it is often a sad mixture of bargaining and denial disguised as spirituality and leads to disappointment and sometimes bitterness. Please don't get me wrong here. Physical healing at God's hand does happen and I've seen it, but probably more in the third world than the first where the media could easily misconstrue it.

As Gail cautioned, *putting one's focus on the physical, takes it off of the spiritual* and that is what matters most to God.

Gail went on, "I have been one who is intense, a perfectionist, and a bit driven. Okay, accelerator to the floorboard. I don't like to control others, but I do like to control me. Oh yes, I love to risk, but only on MY terms. This has accounted for a great deal of inner tension, which over fifty-five years of life, accumulates and doesn't resolve itself. It's more complex, but for me the bottom line is that this cancer brings out in the open all those small and large fears of losing control and it is all symptomatic of a large dose of self-inflicted and enemy induced shame."

"The third verse of *A Mighty Fortress Is Our God*, which speaks of the power and cruelty of Satan, ends with the poignant phrase, 'One little word shall fell him.' That word for me is a gush of cool water poured over one who was weary to the bone of trying; that word is grace. This is what really needed healing now, as the Lord wills; my body is free to follow."

Gale spent the last years of her life building relationships with women all around the world. Through it all, even down the home stretch, she was bursting with joy. She ran so well! I doubt anyone who met her will forget that smile or the Jesus who was behind it. Windrunners are like that.

# Day 5

# A Windrunner's Journal

*I invite you to reread every sentence above which is **bold** and in **italics**. Write it down, in your own words if you wish, to remember it, reflect on it, discuss it, or even memorize it.*

_____

_____

_____

_____

_____

_____

_____

_____

_____

_____

_____

_____

# Time to Write the Rest of Your Life's Script

You are not given the time you have left for your own sake; you have an evangelical mission to become a witness to Hope. You do it best with a changed life. God has revealed something about Himself in your story and He has written your life like a personal letter to your loved ones for whom it will bring special meaning.

God is either in your life or He isn't. *Which is it?*

You have willingly surrendered your heart and soul to Him or not. *Which is it?*

You are letting Him guide and cheer you on or you are not. *Which is it?*

You are either letting Him inspire, educate, bless, rescue, and heal or not. *Which is it?*

Immunity to the fear of death seems entirely mysterious to anyone who doesn't have it. It comes only through the words of the one who has Himself conquered death, Jesus. Go to Him. Receive His words like a transfusion and let them fill you up.

# CONCLUSION

# THE GLORIOUS
# HOME STRETCH

"LIFE SHOULD NOT BE A JOURNEY TO
THE GRAVE WITH THE INTENTION OF
ARRIVING SAFELY IN AN ATTRACTIVE AND
WELL PRESERVED BODY, RATHER TO SKID
IN SIDEWAYS, COVERED IN SCARS, BODY
THOROUGHLY USED UP, TOTALLY WORN
OUT, AND SCREAMING, 'YAHOO , WHAT
A RIDE!'" WHILE EDWARD GRYLLS, BETTER
KNOWN AS BEAR, THE NICKNAME GIVEN
HIM BY HIS SISTER, WAS SPEAKING OF HIS
ADVENTUROUS LIFE TESTING HIS SURVIVAL
SKILLS IN THE WILDERNESS, THIS MAN, OF

A QUIET, BUT SUSTAINING FAITH, COULD HAVE BEEN SPEAKING ABOUT GIVING HIS ALL ON HIS BELL LAP. WE ADMIRE SPORTS TEAMS WHO LEAVE IT ALL ON THE COURT/ TURF IN THEIR LAST GAME. NOW IS OUR CHANCE TO DO THE SAME. **KNOW WHERE YOU ARE GOING**

It matters not so much what is going on in your life as where your life is going. There are many paths and we may stumble or stray. It matters less which path or whether you scuff your knees, but it matters immensely the destination. Fix your eyes on Jesus is the message of the book of Hebrews, the pioneer and perfector of faith who does so despite the travail—all "for the joy set before Him."

Awareness of your destination makes all the difference in how you interpret each step behind and anticipate each step ahead. Wisdom and contentment can grow happily alongside mystery and doubt. Happy steps can bring gratitude and a foretaste of more to come or it can bring a course with the nothingness of "I deserve." Steps of travail can be worth enduring for the sake of final glory (happiness) or they can be bitter injustices of a pointless journey. The former is motivated by hope and the later impaired by fear and each is determined by the destination.

## STEP OUT OF TIME

We live as though we are trapped time and as we head down the home stretch, it seems like the trap is closing. Remember God calls us to join Him beyond time, in the God dimension, even as we live. While the human condition is created in time, it was never intended to be enslaved by it.

Somehow the human experience requires a perception of measure, but it has been adulterated by the human constructs of "not enough" and "I'm gonna miss out" leading to every strife, greed, envy, dissatisfaction, and conflict. They are like slave masters crying hurry, hurry, hurry, more, more, more, I need, I want, I deserve, it's not fair.

Christ's message calls us beyond need and time, "I am sufficient, I will provide, I will complete the good work I've started in you," and with no mention of not enough time or when. For God, time is not an issue. It is not a trap, a constraint or a whip. Perhaps we had to be allowed to experience "not enough" in order to recognize what enough looks like. When we have trusted Him for the little things, we can then trust Him for the big things, step through the looking glass, step through the back of the wardrobe with Lucy, step over the gunwale of the boat with Peter, and fixing our gaze on Jesus, walk, even run down the home stretch.

# Whoever Claims to Live In Him Must Walk As Jesus Did

*We know that we have come to know him if we obey his commands. The man who says I know him, but does not do what he commands is a liar and the truth is not in him. But if anyone obeys his word, God's love is truly made complete in him. This is how we know we are in him: whoever claims to live in him must walk as Jesus did.* (1 John 2:3)

"To know" in the original Greek means more than intellectual knowing. It means a deep intimate connection. It is like the "I see you" of the movie *Avatar*. Out of such a connection with Jesus grows a desire to behave just like Him. If we find our desire waning and our actions falling short, the solution is to go deeper with Christ. This is never truer than when we are coming down the stretch.

> *Whoever claims to live in Jesus must walk as He did including His cross walk: the whole time leading up to His scourging and crucifixion. He knew it was coming and he knew it would be wrought with difficult decisions, unspeakable pain and spiritual anguish – even confusion. That sounds a bit like someone who knows that cancer will take their life. Jesus knew it was not the end of the story – and so must we. Nothing can take from*

*you a life you have already given to Jesus. But that doesn't mean Satan has removed his target from your chest and won't try. So **Stay alert! Watch out for your greatest enemy, the devil. He prowls around like a roaring lion looking for someone to devour. Stand firm against him, and be strong in your faith.** Remember your Christian brothers and sisters all over the world are going through the same kind of suffering you are.*" (1 Peter 5:8)

The enemy knows that if he hasn't got you yet this is his last chance and his quiver is full of arrows named fear, deceit, and deception. You especially need the "full armor of God" to resist him now (Ephesians 6:12).

Jesus asks Peter, "Who do you say I am" (Matthew 16:15, Mark 8:27, Luke 9:18), and agrees with his response, "You're the Christ, the son of the living God" – a divine human being. In His humanness, Jesus knew from Daniel's prophecies that He would be "cut off." He knew He would be rejected and that He would be killed at the hands of His own people. In His divinity, as an inseparable part of the triune God, we can surmise that He knew how and when and why He would die. Yet, while His divinity informed His humanity, it did not immunize Him from the pain and suffering the Father/Son would endure together at Calvary. While He knew He would die an unimaginably horrid death, He walked toward it, not away. He knew the schedule and He submitted to it. Whoever claims to live in Him must walk as Jesus did!

From the time He affirmed His identity as the Christ, "He began explaining to His disciples that He must go to Jerusalem and suffer many things at the hands of the elders, chief priests and teachers of the law, and He must be killed and on the third day be raised to life" (Matthew 16:21). He knows what is coming and yet He walks toward it each day with meaning and purpose. Whoever claims to live in Him must walk as Jesus did!

Peter didn't like to hear what Jesus said, "and began to rebuke him, 'This shall never happen to you'" (Matthew 16:22). You need to be wary of the advice of friends who can easily confuse their hopes for you with God's will for you. As their love and concern is so clearly genuine, it can be tempting to believe their predictions. Christ's response to Peter nails it, "Get behind me, Satan! You are a stumbling block to me; you do not have in mind the things of God, but the things of man" (Matthew 16:23).

## CELEBRATE AND ANTICIPATE – JESUS DID

Only when you have run the backstretch and far corner well in your heart can you cruise down the home stretch. That is what Jesus did. It was biologically arduous, but socially and spiritually rich. Notice what He did before His arrest, conviction, and crucifixion. He celebrated. "My appointed time is near. I'm going to celebrate" (Matthew 26:18). What was He going to celebrate? What God had done. With whom? His dearest friends, the disciples. He anticipated: "that day when I drink it (the fruit of the vine) with you in my father's kingdom" (Matthew 26:29). Start celebrating early and if you have time, do it again. Reread the home stretch chapter in *Cancer's Bell Lap & The Dragon Behind the Door*. Remember that if you put it off you may run out of time and energy to enjoy it – or even worse, miss out altogether on the party at your memorial service after you're gone.

Whoever claims to live in Him must walk as Jesus did. When you do, you will run into the same temptations He did. Look for them. They will be attractive and full of self-interest. Jesus kept walking as He always had—with confidence and purpose. He kept healing and teaching and He started talking about heaven and eternal life. Seek your purpose. Stick with it and start talking about heaven and eternal life. Walk as Jesus did.

The Gospels record that Jesus told His disciples three times explicitly that He was going to die and how, and that He would be raised on the third day. We have a lot in common with them. They didn't get it and we don't either. We haven't needed to, but that all changes when the Bell rings. You had better get it by the time you are rounding the last corner and the finish line is coming into view.

What will you see? Sulfurous fumes rising from a murky chasm or the silhouette of the Father with arms outstretched against a backdrop of dazzling glory? Will you be one of the walking dead now broken to your knees still trying to escape the inexorable conveyor belt dragging you towards the pit? Or will you be racing down the stretch with the crowds cheering, with the wind of the Spirit at your back, leaning on Jesus, your support and pacesetter with your eyes fixed on the Father?

Much of human history is about the intersection and contrasts between the haves and the have-nots, those with guns of steel and those without, those with inherited wealth or without, with education or without. Sometimes it was just about luck. There is no more stark contrast between the haves and the have-nots than down the homestretch: those with Jesus and those without, those with the calm expectant eyes versus those with vacant eyes of resignation and dread. The difference has nothing to do with inheritance or luck. It's all about a choice; and everyone gets one. Remember, I am not speaking from the perspective of a preacher, but as one who has looked into the eyes of countless patients with every sort of malady dying on the cancer wards, in the hospice or their own beds at home. Choose wisely my friend, it makes all the difference.

Living a life of faith by choice demands living by what one cannot see, control or predict. "The transformation of all things occurs where the riddle of human life reaches its culmination point. The hope of His Glory emerges for us when nothing but the existentiality of God remains, and He becomes to us the veritable and living God, whom we can apprehend only as against us stands there—for us."[9] The culmination point is where you discover whether you are a true or false child of God, a charlatan or a crusader, whether your commitment to God is validated or refuted, and whether the ending is happy or hell.

If you have the right stuff, the God stuff, you can be sure there are sons and daughters chasing after you to get it. That's what kids do. If you have taught them well, they will know where it came from and who stood by you through your trials. They will know that it is the only stuff that enables you to run like the wind down the home stretch. Others will catch a glimpse of something special breathed into a home stretch runner and for the very first time recognize it as Jesus.

"To see is to remember!" — Nathan Macuca

Fatigue will be building, muscles aching, breath growing short, and a fragile soul wearing thin. Crowds in the stands will be on their feet, some waving farewell, and others waving welcome, but all cheering. Down the homestretch a runner will be slipping toward that fatal disorientation as their last step breaks through the finish line veil. Of a sudden comes a reassembling of thoughts set free from delirium and movements freed from rigor. With a celestial overture rising and an illusion shattering

---

[9]   Richard Rohr and Joseph Martos, *Wild to Wise*. Franciscan Media. 2005.

light, wonder of wonders, a new life will be beginning. A runner is coming home to new shoes.

Grasp fully how the story ends and let it ignite your passion for running and lighten your load. Then take off running with the wind.

Wendell passed the baton to me. He never told me what to do with it, but he showed me. I got to watch him run with the "breathless expectation" into what lay ahead leaving in his wake blessings and batons well passed, even on the homestretch which ended in victory on April 9, 1987. Now I pass it to you. Run well. Start soon.

## Windrunner Recommendations

- *Start a conversational relationship with Jesus—get to know Him.*
- *Learn His promises and calling for you—try trusting Him.*
- *Practice waiting for His answers—learn to recognize them.*
- *Invest in relationships—build community.*
- *Stock your scripture arsenal and recount your answered prayers—they are your ammunition against the enemy.*
- *Pass every baton you discover—and do it again.*
- *Let the joyful anticipation of God's plans for you deepen, then run with "breathless expectation" into them.*
- *Celebrate it all relationships, memories, experiences—All His Provisions.*

# APPENDIX 1

# GOD'S PROMISES: WEAPONS AND AMMUNITION AGAINST THE DRAGON

*Be strong in the Lord and in his mighty power. Put on the full armor of god so that you can take your stand against the devil's schemes . . .so that when the day of evil comes, you may be able to stand your ground.* (Ephesians 6:10-11)

There is more going on here than it seems and far more than you can handle on your own, in all of life and especially life with cancer. A battle rages in every realm, those you can see and those you can't. All of them: the physical, emotional, social, and spiritual. The devil will use the suffering that is unavoidable in our fallen world to plant seeds of doubt in God in a hurting heart.

> *Stand firm with the belt of truth buckled around your waist, with the breastplate of righteousness in place, and with your feet fitted with the readiness that comes from the gospel of peace. In addition, take up the shield of faith, with which you can extinguish all the flaming arrows of the evil one. Take the helmet of salvation and the sword of the Spirit, which is the word of God. And pray in the spirit on all occasions with all kinds of prayers and requests.* (Ephesians 6:14-18)

You need **protection, confidence, cunning, and weaponry**. God offers them all to those who will appropriate them.

The enemy is real whatever you choose to call it and stalks you 24/7. You need ammunition to take it out, the dragon/devil, along with every one of his deceiving and disconcerting schemes. If equipped, you can walk through any door without fearing what is behind it and sleep through the dark without fearing unseen arrows.

The armor of God's truth is essential, but not enough if it's rusty and stored off in the attic of your memory. A shield slung over your shoulder and sword in its scabbard are not enough.

You need them in a practiced hand raised and coupled with wary eyes scanning the horizons for danger.

In the *BELL LAP and the DRAGON BEHIND THE DOOR*, we spent a lot of time considering all the ways the enemy can come at you with well disguised fears, denials, and bargaining options to alert your eyes. In this book, we have focused on the weaponry in God's armor, His truth, and His promises. Now the focus shifts to using it, hour by hour, day by day. Windrunners are not only equipped and alert, they are also actively engaged on defense – swords unsheathed.

**The first defense is a grateful heart**. We were not born with it. We must cultivate it on our own and muster it daily. Start by first kicking out the dullness and complacency that has crept in like a soggy blanket to smother the wonder you once had as a child. Then awaken yourself to all the things for which you can be grateful, both big and small. Inventory your life before your eyes open on the morning and again after they close at night and follow that with a prayer of thanksgiving. It will get your day off with more strength and your nights with more peace.

Some say "why bother, won't change anything!" but it does. This habit is one thing consistently and totally under your control and can make you genuinely happy. But more than that, a heart filled with gratitude is buffered against the unavoidable bad stuff that inflicts every life. Aggravation and misfortune don't disappear, but are easier to manage. Runners are able to leap higher hurdles when powered by a grateful heart.

**The second defense is to inventory your ammunition** and thereby reestablish your confidence in it. Pull out a few verses and review them. Tape them to your mirror or your refrigerator. Start the day strong. Then carry your weaponry with you, ready to draw at a moment's notice, on flashcards or on your phone, in your purse or your pocket. Be familiar with each one so you can draw the one you need when you need it. It sounds so simple; let its power amaze you.

Finally, **fill your in-between times with God's music**: listen, meditate on the words, hum along and even sing. Without even thinking, certain words will touch your soul and the melody can connect with a place inside that is beyond words. Both can reverberate through those vacant moments which fear loves to invade. Maybe it is even God calling. Maybe it is even Him bringing His protection right to you: He does things like that, and, you will know when it happens - and be glad!

Classic hymns and contemporary worship music are alike in authorship. They have both been written by real people who have encountered God, usually in the depths of life's valleys and bled their experiences into prose. They are often people at the point of giving up who didn't, people without enough strength or purpose who found them. Listen long enough and you are likely to hear a kindred soul singing your life. Listen long enough and you will hear much of God's truth and promises lifted right out of Scripture and put to music.

Below are such verses collated by Dave and several other Windrunners. They took them everywhere they went and some memorized their favorites. They were prepared. They pulled them out whenever a black cloud appeared or a door knob felt hot. Collect those that speak to you and let them grow your confidence, lighten your load, and inspire anticipation for what God has planned.

## GOD'S PROMISES

**His Love in John 3:16-18** - "This is how much God loved the world: He gave his Son, his one and only Son. And this is why: so that no one need be destroyed; by believing in him, anyone can have a whole and lasting life. God didn't go to all the trouble of sending his Son merely to point an accusing finger, telling the world how bad it was. He came to help, to put the world right again. Anyone who trusts in him is acquitted; anyone who refuses to trust him has long since been under the death sentence without knowing it. And why? Because of that person's failure to believe in the one-of-a-kind Son of God when introduced to him" (MSG).

**The Reality, Not the Illusion in 1 John 5:11-15** – "My purpose in writing is simply this: that you who believe in God's Son will know beyond the shadow of a doubt that you have eternal life, the reality and not the illusion. And how bold and free we then become in his presence, freely asking according to his will, sure that he's listening. And if we're confident that he's listening, we know that what we've asked for is as good as ours" (MSG).

***Come near to God and He will come near to you*** in James 4:8.

**Healing in James 5:16** – "Therefore confess your sins to each other and pray for each other so that you may be healed. The prayer of a righteous person is powerful and effective."

**Eternal Life in 2 Peter 1:5-11** - "For this very reason, make every effort to add to your faith goodness; and to goodness, knowledge; and to knowledge, self-control; and to self-control, perseverance; and to perseverance, godliness; and to godliness, mutual affection; and to mutual affection, love...For if you do these things, you will never stumble, and you will receive a rich welcome into the eternal kingdom of our Lord and Savior Jesus Christ."

**Salvation of Your Soul in 1 Peter 1:8-9** – "Though you have not seen him, you love him; and even though you do not see him now, you believe in him and are filled with an inexpressible and glorious joy, for you are receiving the end result of your faith, the salvation of your souls."

**Confidence in Him and His Plan in Philippians 1:6** – "Being confident of this, that he who began a good work in you will carry it on to completion until the day of Christ Jesus."

## He Is There for You in Psalm 91 -

*Whoever dwells in the shelter of the Most High*
*will rest in the shadow of the Almighty.*
*I will say of the LORD, "HE IS MY REFUGE AND MY FORTRESS,*
*my God, in whom I trust."*
*Surely he will save you*
*from the fowler's snare*
*and from the deadly pestilence.*
*He will cover you with his feathers,*
*and under his wings you will find refuge;*
*his faithfulness will be your shield and rampart.*
*You will not fear the terror of night,*
*nor the arrow that flies by day,*
*nor the pestilence that stalks in the darkness,*
*nor the plague that destroys at midday.*
*A thousand may fall at your side,*
*ten thousand at your right hand,*
*but it will not come near you.*
*You will only observe with your eyes*
*and see the punishment of the wicked.*
*If you say, "The LORD IS MY REFUGE,"*
*and you make the Most High your dwelling,*
*no harm will overtake you,*
*no disaster will come near your tent.*
*For he will command his angels concerning you*

> *to guard you in all your ways;*
>
> *they will lift you up in their hands,*
>
> *so that you will not strike your foot against a stone.*
>
> *You will tread on the lion and the cobra;*
>
> *you will trample the great lion and the serpent.*
>
> *"Because he loves me," says the* LORD*, "I* WILL RESCUE HIM*;*
>
> *I will protect him, for he acknowledges my name.*
>
> *He will call on me, and I will answer him;*
>
> *I will be with him in trouble,*
>
> *I will deliver him and honor him.*
>
> *With long life I will satisfy him*
>
> *and show him my salvation."*

**Death Is Gone for Good in Revelation 21:3-5** - "I heard a voice thunder from the Throne: "Look! Look! God has moved into the neighborhood, making his home with men and women! **They're his people, he's their God. He'll wipe every tear from their eyes. Death is gone for good—tears gone, crying gone, pain gone—all the first order of things gone."** The Enthroned continued, "Look! I'm making everything new. Write it all down—each word dependable and accurate" (MSG emphasis added).

**You Will Find Rest in Matthew 11:29** – "Take my yoke upon you and learn from me, for I am gentle and humble in heart, and you will find rest for your souls."

**Afflictions Now Mean Eternal Glory Later in 2 Corinthians 4:17-18** – "For our light and momentary troubles are achieving for us an eternal glory that far outweighs them all. So we fix our eyes not on what is seen, but on what is unseen, since what is seen is temporary, but what is unseen is eternal."

**Adoption into His Family in Ephesians 1:4-6** – "Long before he laid down earth's foundations, he had us in mind, had settled on us as the focus of his love, to be made whole and holy by his love. Long, long ago he decided to adopt us into his family through Jesus Christ. (What pleasure he took in planning this!) He wanted us to enter into the celebration of his lavish gift-giving by the hand of his beloved Son" (MSG).

**To Love, to Be Loved in 1 John 4:17-18** – "God is love. When we take up permanent residence in a life of love, we live in God and God lives in us. This way, love has the run of the house, becomes at home and mature in us, so that we're free of worry on Judgment Day—our standing in the world is identical with Christ's. There is no room in love for fear. Well-formed love banishes fear. Since fear is crippling, a fearful life—fear of death, fear of judgment—is one not yet fully formed in love" (MSG).

**New Heaven and a New Earth in 2 Peter 3:13** – "But in keeping with his promise we are looking forward to a new heaven and a new earth, where righteousness dwells."

**He Is Faithful in 1 John 1:8-9** – "If we claim to be without sin, we deceive ourselves and the truth is not in us. If we confess our sins, he is faithful and just and will forgive us our sins and purify us from all unrighteousness."

**He Forgives and Heals in Psalm 103:2-5** - "Praise the LORD, my soul, and forget not all his benefits—who forgives all your sins and heals all your diseases, who redeems your life from the pit and crowns you with love and compassion, who satisfies your desires with good things so that your youth is renewed like the eagle's."

**He Removes Your Transgressions in Psalm 103:8-12** – "The LORD is compassionate and gracious, slow to anger, abounding in love. He will not always accuse, nor will he harbor his anger forever; he does not treat us as our sins deserve or repay us according to our iniquities. For as high as the heavens are above the earth, so great is his love for those who fear him; as far as the east is from the west, so far has he removed our transgressions from us."

**He Will Direct Your Path in Proverbs 3:5-6** – "Trust in the **LORD** WITH ALL YOUR HEART, AND LEAN NOT ON YOUR OWN UNDERSTANDING; IN ALL YOUR WAYS SUBMIT TO HIM, AND HE WILL MAKE YOUR PATHS STRAIGHT."

**He Works All Things for Our Good in Romans 8:28** – "And we know that in all things God works for the good of those who love him, who have been called according to his purpose. Meanwhile, the moment we get tired in the waiting, God's Spirit is right alongside helping us along. If we don't know how or what to pray, it doesn't matter. He does our praying in and for us, making prayer out of our wordless sighs, our aching groans. He knows us far better than we know ourselves, knows our pregnant condition, and keeps us present before God. That's why we can be so sure that every detail in our lives of love for God is worked into something good" (MSG).

## CONCERNING THE RACE

**Hebrews 12:1 says,** "Therefore, since we are surrounded by such a great cloud of witnesses, let us throw off everything that hinders and the sin that so easily entangles. And let us run with perseverance the race marked out for us."

**1 Corinthians 9:24 says,** "Do you not know that in a race all the runners run, but only one gets the prize? Run in such a way as to get the prize.

**Isaiah 40:28-31 says,** "Do you not know? Have you not heard? The LORD IS THE EVERLASTING GOD, THE CREATOR OF THE ENDS OF THE EARTH. HE WILL NOT GROW TIRED OR WEARY, AND HIS UNDERSTANDING NO ONE CAN FATHOM. HE GIVES STRENGTH TO THE WEARY AND INCREASES THE POWER OF THE WEAK. Even youths grow tired and weary, and young men stumble and fall; but those who hope in the LORD WILL RENEW THEIR STRENGTH. THEY WILL SOAR ON WINGS LIKE EAGLES; THEY WILL RUN AND NOT GROW WEARY, THEY WILL WALK AND NOT BE FAINT."

**2 Timothy 4:7 says,** "I have fought the good fight, I have finished the race, I have kept the faith."

Or,

"You take over. I'm about to die, my life an offering on God's altar. This is the only race worth running. I've run hard right to the finish, believed all the way. All that's left now is the shouting—God's applause! Depend on it, he's an honest judge. He'll do right not only by me, but by everyone eager for his coming" (MSG).

## Concerning Victory

**Philippians 1:21 says,** "For to me, to live is Christ and to die is gain."

**1 Corinthians 15:54 says,** "When the perishable has been clothed with the imperishable, and the mortal with immortality, then the saying that is written will come true: Death has been swallowed up in victory."

**1 Corinthians 16:13 says,** "Be on your guard; stand firm in the faith; be courageous; be strong."

## Peace and Comfort

**Philippians 4:6-7 says,** "Do not be anxious about anything, but in every situation, by prayer and petition, with thanksgiving, present your requests to God. And the peace of God, which transcends all understanding, will guard your hearts and your minds in Christ Jesus."

**Isaiah 26:3 says,** "You will keep in perfect peace those whose minds are steadfast, because they trust in you."

**Psalm 23:4 says,** "Even though I walk through the *valley of the shadow of death* I will fear no evil for you are with me; your rod and your staff, they comfort me."

**Psalm 56:3 says,** "When I am afraid, I put my trust in you. In God, whose word I praise—in God I trust and am not afraid."

**Psalm 27:1, 13-14 says,** "The LORD IS MY LIGHT AND MY SALVATION— WHOM SHALL I FEAR? THE LORD IS THE STRONGHOLD OF MY LIFE— OF WHOM SHALL I BE AFRAID? ...I REMAIN CONFIDENT OF THIS: I WILL SEE THE GOODNESS OF THE LORD IN THE LAND OF THE LIVING. WAIT FOR THE LORD; BE STRONG AND TAKE HEART AND WAIT FOR THE LORD."

**Philippians 4:6-7 says,** "Don't fret or worry. Instead of worrying, pray. Let petitions and praises shape your worries into prayers, letting God know your concerns. Before you know it, a sense of God's wholeness, everything coming together for good, will come and settle you down. It's wonderful what happens when Christ displaces worry at the center of your life" (MSG).

## ENDURANCE

**2 Corinthians 4:10 says,** "We've been surrounded and battered by troubles, but we're not demoralized; we're not sure what to do, but we know that God knows what to do; we've been spiritually terrorized, but God hasn't left our side; we've been thrown down, but we haven't broken. What they did to Jesus, they do to us—trial and torture, mockery and murder; what Jesus did among them, he does in us—he lives! Our lives are at constant risk for Jesus' sake, which makes Jesus' life all the more evident in us. While we're going through the worst, you're getting in on the best!" (MSG).

**2 Corinthians 1:8 says,** "It was so bad we didn't think we were going to make it. We felt like we'd been sent to death row, and that it was all over for us. As it turned out, it was the best thing that could have happened. Instead of trusting in our own strength or wits to get out of it, we were forced to trust God totally—not a bad idea since he's the God who raises the dead! And he did it, rescued us from certain doom. *And* he'll do it again, rescuing us as many times as we need rescuing. You and your prayers are part of the rescue operation" (MSG).

**James 1:2 says,** "Consider it a sheer gift, friends, when tests and challenges come at you from all sides. You know that under pressure, your faith-life is forced into the open and shows its true colors. So don't try to get out of anything prematurely. Let it do its work so you become mature and well-developed, not deficient in any way" (MSG).

# APPENDIX 2

# Mourning – A Necessary Step in Healing

### 1) You Have Got to Do It or It Will Do You

*For sighing comes to me instead of food; my groans*
*pour out like water. I have no peace, no quiet this;*
*I have no rest, but only turmoil.* (Job 3:24, 26)

Loss is an inevitable and universal part of the human experience and mourning it is a natural and indispensable response when you realize what cancer can take from you. Unresolved grief is cumulative and impairs your capacity for healing and happiness.

Many say that grief will simply have its way with you, coming at you when least expected and knocking you over backwards, and that only the passage of time, the fading of memory, and the dulling of senses will bring relief. Others, who have also been there, say that confronting it can cut it down to size and lessen its blows. They assert that while it destroys some hopes it cannot destroy all hope and that actively pursuing new hopes can assuage the loss of the old ones making recovery more possible, although never easy.

No human can tell you how to deal with the unspeakable dismay of a cancer diagnosis or the losses it brings, but God can. The world will try, but the experiences of others who were guided by God may be more helpful. It may require getting past one's anger with God and that needs to be expressed in order to get past it. He is listening and He can handle it. When pain makes it hard to hear His voice, perhaps God can speak through others or even into your own words as you pour your heart out to them.

Grief never leaves, but if you can cut it down to size, heal much of it, and you can learn to live with the rest. It takes an active process of acknowledging what is lost and mourning it. Some suggest that with God grief is unnecessary and unrighteous, not characteristic of someone who really walks with God. That is not true. The Lord has not only granted permission, but welcomes every out-pouring of every heart in every situation. Job's story teaches us that it is okay to despise our disease and the predicament it puts us in, at least for season.

## 2) **Accept the Loss**

Recovery involves improving your ability to embrace the truth and a new future with the new enduring purpose that is not a charade. It's not about acting a particular way, "recovered." "We all want the approval of those around us and because we're tired of feeling bad, we can opt for 'Academy Award' recovery and begin to act recovered even though we are not."[1] Those who perpetually do that act never do their real grieving, never recover, and become trapped in the quiet desperation of their emotions, never able to return to happiness. Unresolved grief is like a ticking time bomb that can explode with outbursts of anger, binge purchasing, overeating, drinking, drugs, and destroyed relationships.

Some need to protect themselves and others with the act so they can grieve in controlled circumstances while also reinventing their lives and discovering new sources of hope and purpose. That can work especially for those who have dependents who will be better able to cope with the circumstances under the tutelage of a recovered patient.

Recovery involves gaining awareness of loss, acknowledging it, and taking responsibility for dealing with it. Surrender some of your other commitments to make space in your life to do it gently.

Recovery is not burying feelings, replacing the loss with a substitute, grieving alone, just giving it time, dwelling on regrets, or losing trust in God's love and plan for you. Acceptance is only possible after doing the painful work that grief requires. You can't go around it or over it, you have got to go through it. Start as soon as you're able to pull the pain out of the closet little by little, face it, deal with some of it, and then put it away until next time. Probably easier said than done, but is possible. Every bit you deal with takes away some of grief's power that the Dragon would love to use to disable you.

The key is to go through your "grief story" with someone safe you can trust who can validate it in gently embrace it with you. It needs a respectful place to reside integrated into your whole life story: what happened is awful, you're not crazy or weak – and you are not alone. We will be your tribe, your village to help you get through the pain.

Not everyone has a friend who can really fill this role, but everyone can find counselor. Find one. Do the work. Embrace the healing. You deserve it.

When your grief has an honorable place to rest, you can pick it up whenever you need to remember and in time even learn and grow through it.

To give up any part of your life is hard because you are still in it, but not really. It is essential because you're losing it, but not quite yet. It's hard because society doesn't teach us how to surrender; it teaches us how to acquire and hold on the things. Recovery requires letting go of the past, even the present, and finding a new meaning for living and a new purpose. That is where God comes in.

**Purpose redefined is often the best bridge to acceptance.**

"I'm going to beat this thing" is often the most available new purpose, but it is not entirely in your control whereas focusing on your baton pass and spiritual journey is. You are strong enough for both with God on your side.

**Acceptance won't take away the hurt, but it will open a door to a new life and that can.**

3) **Act**

Confronting the loss of a planned future is never easy, but always necessary before you can enjoy inventing a new one and you can't do it alone.

Find a safe audience for your story, someone who can validate it. "Yeah, that really sucks!" Take them with you as you seek out and acknowledge your wounds, recognize how they have influenced you, and the mark they have left. It must be a trustworthy friend or counselor with whom you can emotionally express your grief without the fear of driving them away. Often someone who has experienced intense emotional loss themselves is best.

4) **Guard Yourself**

Get lots of rest and don't overextend yourself. Don't take on many new responsibilities or big decisions. Get some exercise and pamper yourself a little. Be sure to schedule time with significant others. Keep a journal periodically and make appointments with it. It is part of pampering yourself to make time for reflection in an environment you like with a companionable cup of coffee or tea. Request a back rub or get a massage. Take hot baths. Go to the sun and watch cheerful movies. Under indulge in the coping mechanisms of our society that can be addictive like drugs, junk food, TV, and tobacco. A little can numb the pain, but only temporarily and a lot can make a little depression worse and disabling.

Know that healing has progressions and regressions and don't let that discourage you. It's okay to feel depressed, crying is a natural release which we are given for a reason. Use it when it calls to you then put it away. Don't stay with it. It's okay to need comforting and to seek the support of others but remember healing is your project and they can't do it for you.

You are the architect of your own discomfort and you need to accept responsibility for your feelings before you can change them. What ruins a picnic? Is it the rain or is it one's attitude towards the rain? Blaming cancer gets you nowhere but helpless and unhappy.

If your past hurts, wash it in forgiveness and choose to not let it define you, then move on. Confess what you needed and longed for, but did not get and what you didn't deserve, but did get. Then choose to not let those define you and move on. When another person was involved, seek to understand their wounds and their perspectives as well as your own. Time for bickering and accusing is gone. Then give each of you a healthy dose of grace and forgiveness and move on.

Mourning can draw you toward God, but blaming God drives you away and leaves you nowhere to turn. Blaming anyone or anything never leads to healing and without that you are only left with a bundle of grief which festers forever.

If you don't have a friend that you can very intentionally do this with, then find a counselor. Invest in yourself and spend time with them. Your goal is to get passed the past and find what you can be grateful for so you can get on with celebrating it. Illness may take away a part of your life, but it also gives you a chance to abandon parts that you simply have accumulated. It gives you a chance to choose the new life you will lead and the new purpose you will serve. **Let the trauma you mourn, begin the transformation you seek.**

> *"No, that trauma you faced was not easy*
> *And God wept that it hurt you so;*
> *But it was allowed to shape your heart*
> *So that into his likeness you'd grow."* [2]
> By Russell Keffer

If you wish to learn more about grief recovery, consultant the *Grief Recovery Handbook*, The Grief Recovery Institute, 8306 Wilshire Blvd., #21 – a, Los Angeles, CA 90211.

# APPENDIX 3

# WHAT WILL HEAVEN BE LIKE AND OTHER QUESTIONS?

Remember: What was written with imagination must be interpreted with imagination. Recognize that because God is doing His best within the limitations of our minds and imaginations, we must not limit Him further by not using them.

## WHAT WILL WE BE IN HEAVEN?

Today my friend Ken carries his quadriplegic wife, Joni Earickson Tada, from their car to her wheelchair and back just as he did many years ago on their first date. I can hardly imagine what it will be like for them to play and dance together in heaven someday. Joni says, "I still can't hardly believe it. I, with shriveled, bent fingers, atrophied muscles, gnarled knees, and no feeling from the shoulders down, will one day have a new body, light, bright, and clothed in righteousness – powerful and dazzling. Can you imagine the hope this gives someone spinal – cord injured like me? Or someone who is cerebral palsied, brain injured or who has multiple sclerosis? Imagine the hope this gives someone who is manic- depressive." **No other religion, no other philosophy promises new bodies, hearts and minds. Only in the gospel of Christ do hurting people find such incredible hope."** (*Heaven: Your Real Home*, Joni Earickson Tada, Grand Rapids: Zondervan, 1995.)

I too look forward to skiing and climbing again with my paraplegic son John, and to renewed intellectual and comedic banter with my schizophrenic son, Max.

Tom and Bill, both in their eighties and both riddled with cancer got to know each other lying side by side in our hospice. Both were bedridden but still able to carry on animated conversations. They knew Jesus and often spoke about heaven and joked about what the fishing and golf would be like and who would get there first.

It seemed Bill might pass at any moment, but he was waiting for his son to arrive from out of town. One morning I arrived to find Bill alone and Tom's bed empty. Bill related that he had had a dream that night that Tom was dying and was calling to him to come along. In his dream he saw Tom walking away framed against a light at the end of a long dark tunnel carrying his fishing pole in one hand and beckoning with the other. Bill said he was so temped to go, but had to wait for his son. Later I learned his son had arrived later that morning and Bill departed shortly after their visit.

Some folks discovered angels sitting on their bed or standing beside them or hovering in the eaves of their room. Sometimes it happened night after night and other times during the day, sometimes only a visible presence and other times with words, but always bringing comfort.

I told you earlier of Al singing to Mary about Heaven as she floated between delirium and rapture. When the tears let up and with the twinkle back in his eye, Al then brought us back to earth half joking with a 98 percent serious question, "Yeah, but there is no marriage in heaven." Implicit in his words "and none of the tenderness, bliss, and ecstatic joy we have known together" and being a guy "no sex either." Being a guy, I thought about that, too. Jesus' words explicitly tell us there will be no marriage (Matthew 22:30) but are silent on sex.

Being a doc, I am accustomed to being the go-to-for-an-swers-guy even on subjects not covered in med school. So, I went prayerfully scrambling for a meaningful response for his question. I went to the textbook of our lives where it seems God so often plants clues for those of us with scriptural knowledge deficiency. The inspiration that came seemed apt for them. Mary is a foodie and gourmet cook and Al is a guy who loves to eat: "When we were kids, you remember how much we loved Mac & Cheese.

There just wasn't anything better. We could eat it every night given the chance. But now as adults there are lots of foods that surpass it. I suspect sex is the Mac & Cheese of this life, while important, it is only a foretaste of something better to come."

For marriage we need to shift from the gastronomic to the psychosocial, from the pursuit of satiety to our intrinsic need for emotional and physical intimacy. Scripture shows us in (Genesis 2:18) that God created us for relationship and that the special relationship He designed in marriage foreshadows a profound mystery, the relationship of Christ to His church (Ephesians 15:31-32). Marriage and the sex that goes with it which having fulfilled its purpose of metaphorically informing us of our coming relationship with Christ and will end. There is no suggestion that our intimate marital relationships will end. There is every suggestion that relationships will continue to grow (1 Thessalonians 4:14-18, Matthew 6:19 -20).

Sex is another matter. C. S. Lewis crafts the explanation in metaphor, "I think our present outlook might be like that of a small boy who, on being told that the sexual act was the highest bodily pleasure should immediately ask whether you ate chocolates at the same time. On receiving the answer 'No,' he might regard absence of chocolates as the chief characteristic of sexuality. In vain would you tell him that the reason why lovers in their carnal raptures don't bother about chocolates is that they have something better to think of. The boy knows chocolate: he does not know the positive thing that excludes it. We are in the same position. We know the sexual life; we do not know, except in glimpses, the other thing for which, in Heaven, we may abandon it

Some speculate that sexual differences will be transcended in heaven in favor of some unisex androgynous hybrid form. I suspect it is more as pastor and novelist Randy Alcorn puts it through the mouthpiece of a fictional angel, Zor, speaking to the story's protagonist about manhood in Heaven "you are like us in that you do not marry or bear children here ( in Heaven), but as for your being a man, what else would you be? Elyon (God) may unmake what men make, but he does not unmake what he makes. He made you male, as he made your mother, wife, and daughters female. Gender is not merely a component of being to be added in or extracted and discarded. It is an essential part of who you are." (*DEADLINE, Sisters*, Ore: Multnomah, 1994, 238).

Similarly, Paul's words in Galatians speak of relational equality in Christ not as an equivalency in anatomy and physiology: "in Christ's family there can be no division into Jew and no Jew, slave and free, male and female. Among us you are all equal. That is, we are all in a common relationship Christ" (Galatians 3:28 MSG).

## NEW EARTH

New Earth will look a lot like the old, not so much different as it is better: plants and trees, mountains and streams, animals and pets, but no pollution, erosion or deforestation. "And of course it is different as a real thing is different from its shadow or as waking is from a dream" (C S Lewis, *The Last Battle,* New York: Collier Books, 19560169-171).

Sadly, we are too often dismissive of the glory of God's creation which we now inhabit. It is exploding all around us both in the natural wonders of the ages and in the wonders of each new spring and new life. Until we can overcome our "take-it-for-grantedness" we cannot set free a "marvel–at-it-allness" which would make it easier to imagine what the Creator has yet in store for us, not just tomorrow but across the great divide. These wonders are not illusions, but for those too blind to see them, they may as well be. If they are illusions, then they are also powerless to be what they are meant to be: a tantalizing foretaste of what is to come!

"The kingdom of heaven is like a treasure hidden in a field, which a man found and covered up. Then in his joy he goes and sells all that he has and buys that field" (Matthew 13:44).

So "if we are exiles and refugees on earth (1 Peter 2:11), and if our citizenship is in heaven (Philippians 3:20), and if nothing can separate us from the love of Christ (Romans 8:35), and if His steadfast love is better than life (Psalm 63:3), and if all hardship is working for us an eternal weight of glory (2 Corinthians 4:17), then we (ought to) give to the winds our fears and "seek first the kingdom of God and his righteousness' (Matthew 6:33)."

Be on your guard though ere the blessings of this world or the next ever take your attention off of Christ, the author and essence of them all. They are the blood-bought evidence of Christ's love, but only a glimpse into the triune God themselves.

C.S. Lewis illustrates what I mean by an experience he had: "I was standing today in the dark tool shed. The sun was shining outside and through the crack at the top of the door there came a sunbeam. From where I stood that beam of light, with the specks of dust floating in it, was the most striking thing in the place. Everything else was almost pitch-black. I was seeing the beam, not seeing the things by it. Then I moved, so that the beam fell on my eyes. Instantly the whole previous picture vanished. I saw no tool shed. And (above all) no beam. Instead I saw, framed in the irregular cranny at the top of the door, green leaves moving on the branches of a tree outside and beyond that, ninety-odd million miles away, the sun. Looking along the beam and looking at the beam are very different experiences." (C.L. Lewis: Meditation in a Toolshed," in C. S. Lewis: *Essay Collection and other Short Pieces,* London: Harper Collins, 2000, 607)

The sunbeams of blessings in our lives and in heaven are bright in and of themselves and they give light to the ground on which we walk and inspiration to our dreams, but there is a higher purpose for these blessings. God means for us to do more than stand outside them and admire them for what they are. Even more, He means for us to walk into them and see the sun from which they come. If the beams are beautiful, the Son is even more beautiful. God's aim is not that we merely admire His gifts, but even more, His glory (paraphrased with apologies to John Piper, *Don't Waste Your Life*, Crossway Books, Wheaton, Illinois. P58).

## BEAM ME UP, SCOTTY

"So if heaven is so great, Doc, why don't you just give me a pill or shot or something and send me on my way. My life is finished here. I'm never going to get better. I can't ski. I can't go to work. I can't make love to my wife or toss the football my son – just give me something. I'm ready."

Jason was in his forties. Sarcoma had destroyed his leg and filled his lungs. He had months to live, not years. I could totally identify with what he was thinking and feeling. I told him that if that was his choice, I was sure there was someone out there who would help him and even encourage him to take his life, but I couldn't because I believed God still had plans for him.

"That's bull, Doc!" he replied and so began a long discussion over weeks then months. It started with suggesting to him that the reason for living wasn't about him, it was about his son, his family, the generations to come, some people he hadn't even met yet, and it was about God. (remember the twin commandments: Love God and love your neighbor)We didn't talk about that at first nor did we talk about how it would be partly about him as well because I knew, as he fulfilled his purpose for them, something mysterious and wonderful was going to happen in him and it did, but he wasn't ready or able to grasp that yet.

Years ago, a proposition came before the voters in Washington State to allow physician-assisted suicide for those with terminal illness. Had I been confronted with that issue years earlier as an intellectual and pragmatic student, I would have supported it. By the time the proposition came up, I had witnessed the lives of countless dying patients and had seen amazing things happen in and through them as they walked through the "valley of the shadow of death" – precious things that would have been a tragedy to have missed. Suffering can deceive us by focusing all of our attention inward. But there is no time in life when Rick Warren's words "it's not about you" are more true. It is really about God and what He has for you and what He has for others through you.

The apostle Paul got it. Despite years in prison, despite misery, uncertainty, loneliness, and despite the excitement of joining Jesus in Heaven after death, he wrote to the Philippians, "because of what you are going through, I'm sure that it is better for me to stick it out here" (Philippians 1:24 MSG). "But it is more necessary for you that I remain in the body" – to go on living for their sake. He recognized that there was a purpose in his suffering "there's far more to this life and trusting Christ. There is also suffering for him but not just for the sake of suffering. The suffering is as much a gift as the trusting" (Philippians 1:29 MSG). Paul is not exulting pain and suffering, but rather Christ who empowers the sufferer to meaningfully endure. Again Paul gets it, "on the contrary, everything happening to me in this jail only serves to make Christ more accurately known... They (the Romans), the prison, the illness, didn't shut me up; they gave me a pulpit! Alive, I am Christ's messenger."

*It's not about you. It's about others. You have a pulpit, probably the highest and most prominent of your lifetime. Don't abdicate it. Show up. Speak boldly. They are all listening.*

## CROSSING THE DIVIDE/HEAVEN'S DOORSTEPS

As we sleep, our subconscious is alive in our dreams. When the alarm rudely goes off the dreams, no matter how animated, end. They die unfinished as reality bursts in. Sometimes as our consciousness is booting up we linger on the threshold of consciousness, one foot holding back anchored in the dream and the other stepping outward with growing awareness of cozy sheets and the glow of a breaking dawn. Then we let go the dream and shake off the stiffness of the nocturnal rigors with a stretch and a yawn to greet a new day and real life. I suspect shaking off rigor mortis and stepping into heaven isn't much different: reluctance and expectation. "Even if a lovely caressing hand is waking us up . . . We only experience it as an intrusion upon the world of our dreams as we attempt to finish them off. Likewise, more often than not death appears to be something dreadful, and we hardly suspect how well it is meant . . .." (Victor Frankle)

# WHAT ABOUT THE LITTLE CHILDREN?

Dallas Willard, professor of theology at the University of California and author of groundbreaking books *The Divine Conspiracy* and many others writes in his last book, *The Allure of Gentleness*, the best and most succinct answer to that poignant question: "The child who dies during a famine (or any illness or accident) is ushered immediately into the full world of God in which he or she finds existence good and prospects incomprehensibly grand. There God is seen, as He now surely is not seen, to be good and great without limit, and every individual received into His presence enjoys the everlasting sufficiency of His goodness and greatness. There is no tragedy for those who rely on this God."

# APPENDIX 4

# WHAT SCRIPTURE SAYS ABOUT HEAVEN

1) **2 Peter 3:13 says,** "But in keeping with his promise we are looking forward to a new heaven and a new earth, where righteousness dwells."

2) **Isaiah 65:17-19 says,** "See, I will create new heavens and a new earth. The former things will not be remembered, nor will they come to mind...the sound of weeping and of crying will be heard in it no more."

3) **Romans 6:23 says,** "For the wages of sin is death, but the gift of God is eternal life in Christ Jesus our Lord."

4) **Romans 3:22-25 says,** "This righteousness is given through faith in Jesus Christ to all who believe. There is no difference between Jew and Gentile, [23] for all have

sinned and fall short of the glory of God, and all are justified freely by his grace through the redemption that came by Christ Jesus. God presented Christ as a sacrifice of atonement, through the shedding of his blood—to be received by faith. He did this to demonstrate his righteousness, because in his forbearance he had left the sins committed beforehand unpunished."

5) **Matthew 6:19-20 says,** "Do not store up for yourselves treasures on earth, where moths and vermin destroy, and where thieves break in and steal. But store up for yourselves treasures in heaven, where moths and vermin do not destroy, and where thieves break in and steal."

6) **Luke 23:43 says,** "Jesus answered him (the criminal on the adjacent cross who recognized Jesus as the Son of God), 'Truly I tell you, today you will be with me in paradise.'"

7) **Revelation 21:1-3 says,** "Then I saw a new heaven and a new earth, for the first heaven and the first earth had passed away, And I heard a loud voice from the throne saying, 'Look! God's dwelling place is now among the people, and he will dwell with them. They will be his people, and God himself will be with them and be their God.'"

8) **Revelation 22:1-5 says,** "Then the Angel showed me Water-of-Life River, crystal bright. It flowed from the Throne of God and the Lamb, right down the middle

of the street. The Tree of Life was planted on each side of the River, producing twelve kinds of fruit, a ripe fruit each month. The leaves of the Tree are for healing the nations. Never again will anything be cursed. The Throne of God and of the Lamb is at the center. His servants will offer God service—worshiping, they'll look on his face, their foreheads mirroring God. Never again will there be any night. No one will need lamplight or sunlight. The shining of God, the Master, is all the light anyone needs. And they will rule with him age after age after age" (MSG).

9) **2 Peter 3:10 says,** "But the day of the Lord will come like a thief. The heavens will disappear with a roar; the elements will be destroyed by fire, and the earth and everything done in it will be laid bare."

10) **1 Corinthians 15:35-41 says**, "But someone will ask, "How are the dead raised? With what kind of body will they come?" How foolish! What you sow does not come to life unless it dies. When you sow, you do not plant the body that will be, but just a seed, perhaps of wheat or of something else. But God gives it a body as he has determined, and to each kind of seed he gives its own body. Not all flesh is the same: People have one kind of flesh, animals have another, birds another and fish another. There are also heavenly bodies and there are earthly bodies; but the splendor of the heavenly bodies

is one kind, and the splendor of the earthly bodies is another. The sun has one kind of splendor, the moon another and the stars another; and star differs from star in splendor.

11) Romans 8:18 says, "I consider that our present sufferings are not worth comparing with the glory that will be revealed in us."

12) Romans 8:19-25 says, "That's why I don't think there's any comparison between the present hard times and the coming good times. The created world itself can hardly wait for what's coming next. Everything in creation is being more or less held back. God reins it in until both creation and all the creatures are ready and can be released at the same moment into the glorious times ahead. Meanwhile, the joyful anticipation deepens. All around us we observe a pregnant creation. The difficult times of pain throughout the world are simply birth pangs. But it's not only around us; it's *within* us. The Spirit of God is arousing us within. We're also feeling the birth pangs. These sterile and barren bodies of ours are yearning for full deliverance. That is why waiting does not diminish us; any more than waiting diminishes a pregnant mother. We are enlarged in the waiting. We, of course, don't see what is enlarging us. But the longer we wait, the larger we become, and the more joyful our expectancy" (MSG).

13) Luke 24:37-39 says, "They were startled and frightened, thinking they saw a ghost. He said to them, "Why are you troubled, and why do doubts rise in your minds? Look at my hands and my feet. It is I myself! Touch me and see; a ghost does not have flesh and bones, as you see I have."

14) Revelation 21:4 says, "He will wipe every tear from their eyes. There will be no more death or mourning or crying or pain, for the old order of things has passed away."

15) Romans 6:23 says, "For the wages of sin is death, but the gift of God is eternal life in[a] Christ Jesus our Lord."

16) Matthew 20:1-16 says in the Parable of the Workers in the Vineyard, "For the kingdom of heaven is like a landowner who went out early in the morning to hire workers for his vineyard. He agreed to pay them a denarius for the day and sent them into his vineyard. About nine in the morning he went out and saw others standing in the marketplace doing nothing. He told them, 'You also go and work in my vineyard, and I will pay you whatever is right.' So they went. He went out again about noon and about three in the afternoon and did the same thing. About five in the afternoon he went out and found still others standing around. He asked them, 'Why have you been standing here all day long doing nothing?' 'Because no one has hired us,' they answered. He said to them, 'You also go and work in my vineyard.' When evening came,

the owner of the vineyard said to his foreman, 'Call the workers and pay them their wages, beginning with the last ones hired and going on to the first.' The workers who were hired about five in the afternoon came and each received a denarius. So when those came who were hired first, they expected to receive more. But each one of them also received a denarius. When they received it, they began to grumble against the landowner. 'These who were hired last worked only one hour,' they said, 'and you have made them equal to us who have borne the burden of the work and the heat of the day.' But he answered one of them, 'I am not being unfair to you, friend. Didn't you agree to work for a denarius? Take your pay and go. I want to give the one who was hired last the same as I gave you. Don't I have the right to do what I want with my own money? Or are you envious because I am generous?' So the last will be first, and the first will be last."

17) **1 Corinthians 13:12 says,** "We don't yet see things clearly. We're squinting in a fog, peering through a mist. But it won't be long before the weather clears and the sun shines bright! We'll see it all then, see it all as clearly as God sees us, knowing him directly just as he knows us!" (MSG).

18) **Romans 8:28 says,** "Meanwhile, the moment we get tired in the waiting, God's Spirit is right alongside helping us

along. If we don't know how or what to pray, it doesn't matter. He does our praying in and for us, making prayer out of our wordless sighs, our aching groans. He knows us far better than we know ourselves, knows our pregnant condition, and keeps us present before God. That's why we can be so sure that every detail in our lives of love for God is worked into something good" (MSG).

19) **Matthew 6:25-34 says,** "Therefore I tell you, do not worry about your life,...²⁵⁻²⁶ "If you decide for God, living a life of God-worship, it follows that you don't fuss about what's on the table at mealtimes or whether the clothes in your closet are in fashion. There is far more to your life than the food you put in your stomach, more to your outer appearance than the clothes you hang on your body. Look at the birds, free and unfettered, not tied down to a job description, careless in the care of God. And you count far more to him than birds. Has anyone by fussing in front of the mirror ever gotten taller by so much as an inch? All this time and money wasted on fashion—do you think it makes that much difference? Instead of looking at the fashions, walk out into the fields and look at the wildflowers. They never primp or shop, but have you ever seen color and design quite like it? The ten best-dressed men and women in the country look shabby alongside them. If God gives such attention to the appearance of wildflowers—most of which are

never even seen—don't you think he'll attend to you, take pride in you, do his best for you? What I'm trying to do here is to get you to relax, to not be so preoccupied with *getting,* so you can respond to God's *giving.* People who don't know God and the way he works fuss over these things, but you know both God and how he works. Steep your life in God-reality, God-initiative, God-provisions. Don't worry about missing out. You'll find all your everyday human concerns will be met. Give your entire attention to what God is doing right now, and don't get worked up about what may or may not happen tomorrow. God will help you deal with whatever hard things come up when the time comes" (MSG).

20) **John 14:1-4 says,** "Do not let your hearts be troubled. You believe in God; believe also in me. My Father's house has many rooms; if that were not so, would I have told you that I am going there to prepare a place for you? And if I go and prepare a place for you, I will come back and take you to be with me that you also may be where I am. You know the way to the place where I am going."

21) **Psalm 16:11 says,** "You make known to me the path of life; you will fill me with joy in your presence, with eternal pleasures at your right hand."

22) **1 Corinthians 9:24-27 says,** "Do you not know that in a race all the runners run, but only one gets the prize? Run in such a way as to get the prize. Everyone who competes

in the games goes into strict training. They do it to get a crown that will not last, but we do it to get a crown that will last forever. Therefore I do not run like someone running aimlessly; I do not fight like a boxer beating the air. No, I strike a blow to my body and make it my slave so that after I have preached to others, I myself will not be disqualified for the prize."

23) **Luke 6:21 says,** "Coming down off the mountain with them, he stood on a plain surrounded by disciples, and was soon joined by a huge congregation from all over Judea and Jerusalem, even from the seaside towns of Tyre and Sidon. They had come both to hear him and to be cured of their ailments. Those disturbed by evil spirits were healed. Everyone was trying to touch him—so much energy surging from him, so many people healed! Then he spoke: You're blessed when you've lost it all. God's kingdom is there for the finding. You're blessed when you're ravenously hungry. Then you're ready for the Messianic meal. You're blessed when the tears flow freely. Joy comes with the morning" (MSG).

24) **Luke 24:41-43 says,** "While they were saying all this, Jesus appeared to them and said, "Peace be with you." They thought they were seeing a ghost and were scared half to death. He continued with them, "Don't be upset, and don't let all these doubting questions take over. Look at my hands; look at my feet—it's really me. Touch me.

Look me over from head to toe. A ghost doesn't have muscle and bone like this." As he said this, he showed them his hands and feet. They still couldn't believe what they were seeing. It was too much; it seemed too good to be true. He asked, "Do you have any food here?" They gave him a piece of leftover fish they had cooked. He took it and ate it right before their eyes" (MSG).

25) **Mark 14:25 says,** "Truly I tell you, I will not drink again from the fruit of the vine until that day when I drink it new in the kingdom of God."

26) **Matthew 8:11 says,** "I say to you that many will come from the east and the west, and will take their places at the feast with Abraham, Isaac and Jacob in the kingdom of heaven."

27) **Revelation 21:27 says,** "Nothing impure will ever enter it, nor will anyone who does what is shameful or deceitful, but only those whose names are written in the Lamb's book of life."

28) **1 John 5:11-13 says,** "And this is the testimony: God has given us eternal life, and this life is in his Son. Whoever has the Son has life; whoever does not have the Son of God does not have life. I write these things to you who believe in the name of the Son of God so that you may know that you have eternal life."

29) **John 14:13-14 says,** "And I will do whatever you ask in my name, so that the Father may be glorified in the Son. You may ask me for anything in my name, and I will do it."

30) **2 Timothy 2:11 says,** "Here is a trustworthy saying: If we died with him, we will also live with him."

31) **Colossians 3:3-4 says,** "For you died, and your life is now hidden with Christ in God. 4 When Christ, who is your life, appears, then you also will appear with him in glory."

32) **Luke 22:28-30 says,** "You are those who have stood by me in my trials. And I confer on you a kingdom, just as my Father conferred one on me, so that you may eat and drink at my table in my kingdom and sit on thrones, judging the twelve tribes of Israel."

33) **John 12:25 says,** "Anyone who loves their life will lose it, while anyone who hates their life in this world will keep it for eternal life."

34) **Matthew 10:39 says,** "Whoever finds their life will lose it, and whoever loses their life for my sake will find it."

35) **Hebrews 2:14-15 says,** "Since the children have flesh and blood, he too shared in their humanity so that by his death he might break the power of him who holds the power of death—that is, the devil—and free those who all their lives were held in slavery by their fear of death."

36) **1 Peter 1:3-5 says,** "We've been given.........when you'll have it all- life healed and whole."

# APPENDIX 5

# A SPIRITUAL JOURNEY
# CLIFF NOTES

*"Spirituality is not a private search for what is highest in oneself but a communal search for the face of God. The call of God is double: Worship divinity and link yourself to humanity. There are two great and equal commandments: Love God and love your neighbor."*
*The Holy Longing* by Richard Rohr

## JESUS CHANGES OUR WORLD VIEW

The vision of the world and life that Jesus gives is very different from the worldview we have today. Anyone or anything which has power and control in this world and life has a vested interest in keeping things just as they are and that includes many of us. As death will steal even these from you, you may as well take a look at Jesus' point of view as the Windrunners did.

Their story started with their becoming disciples and "starting to grow in four specific areas: to know Christ, to love Christ, to trust Christ, and to follow Christ,"[1] such that they became more and more like Him. Note obedience is not a requirement, but rather an elective response that grows out of knowing, loving, trusting, and following. Sadly, others who call themselves Christians do those four so poorly that the moniker is misleading and indeed does disservice to Christ. The very sight of some mediocre efforts, both outside and sadly inside the church, can be enough to turn many an observer away. But come inside and join a community of disparate individuals joined most often in a common humble search for God's face.

If you struggle with some aspects of the church, or some people in the church, you're in good company. If it seems at times like the church is off message, abusing power, hypocritical or sidetracked with legalistic quibbling, you share the anger of an itinerant preacher in Palestine 2000 years ago named Jesus. His response was, "Come to Me." Look not, therefore, at our fallible peers, but go directly to Jesus. No intercessor or institution is necessary to endorse or craft your personal journey and relationship with Him. Better to become a follower of Jesus than to just become a Christian and have to contend with all the baggage attached. Instead, wed your soul to His.

## GUARD YOUR HEART

Your heart is vulnerable. The enemy has it in its sights. His quiver is full of deadly arrows, fear, confusion, loneliness, depression, despair, denial, and they are all aimed at your heart. "Above all else, guard your heart, for it is the wellspring of life" (Proverbs 4:23). Cancer will send little messages at you from every direction, stories of others taken out by cancer, stories that say I've got you and you will never be free, I will haunt you all hours of the night and day, and your life will never be good again. All subliminal messages that say now you are irrelevant, without purpose or value. Those are all lies, but if your heart agrees with them, they will take you out.

When you are already overwhelmed, it is easy to let a wet blanket mood of worthlessness and hopelessness settle over you. Toss it off, kick it out, and claim the truths of Scripture: your identity and value are God given and your purposes are God ordained. The enemy can try with cancer to steal or thwart them, but this is where God comes in.

Many say that with God's help you can win this battle and I agree. I'm not talking about treating your disease right now, I'm talking about saving your heart and your life and I'm talking about every time and forever. You have to know who you really are and discover God's purpose for you in spite of cancer in order to run a Bell Lap with the Windrunners – a lap that is meaningful, creative, purposeful and even full of joy and often long. It takes a spiritual journey with Jesus and that is the only effective route to freedom, peace, and power that I have seen. If you're able to do that, then you will also have the best shot at defeating the enemy and controlling your cancer. Imagine that. I know it's true. I have seen it time and again.

God wants your heart. If you let go of it and give it to Him, He will protect it.

I have had people tell me, "Sure that makes sense to get God involved, but it is pretty ridiculous. I can't do that. It would mean giving up hope for survival. I've got to have hope." Yes, hope is essential, but the letting go I am speaking of does not abandon hope. That only happens if you choose defeat in detachment or resignation to become the Walking Dead when you let go of your life without grabbing onto God's promises for you in both this life and the next. You are not abandoning anything but adding something.

## DISSOLUTION?

If you saw a bunch of scrappy kids playing football in the park with imperfect technique, one passing poorly, another dropping the ball, still another cheating, and another throwing punches after the whistle, you wouldn't conclude that football a worthless sport. You would just chalk it up to lack of training, silly pride, and testosterone.

Many Christians who are just learning to follow Christ are still struggling with self-centeredness and are just the same. It is like becoming a football player or a sailor. The decision is made, then one steps on board the ship, but one is not really much of a sailor yet. It takes training and practice. You start feeling how the boat moves under sail, and how it responds to the wind and currents. Then you model the old salts who sense things you can't even see yet. It's an adventure just like learning to understand God and become like Christ.

God's voice can be as soft as a zephyr or as booming as in my bear encounter. Sometimes you have to go to His Word, the Bible, for clarity or take hints coming from His creation. Kelp shows sailors where the reefs are and a blackened sky marks the coming storm. When waves of anxiety rock your soul or blackened spirits mar your relationships, you're seeing the kelp and probably not walking a Christ inspired path and heading for a reef. *It is time to be searching for every way God is trying to communicate with you with* His voice: softly in your heart, boldly in the Bible, or through events or the words of pastors and friends. It takes practice like becoming a sailor. Start soon and practice often.

## QUESTIONS AND ANSWERS

A spiritual journey starts with asking your questions. It is different from joining a religion which provides a template of answers for you to kowtow to. Great harm comes when answers precede questions: Understanding becomes unnecessary and often never sought and without understanding you can become lost in a quagmire when new questions don't fit the old rote answers. Disillusionment and disengagement follow. Don't let them. Ask your own questions and go after understanding your own answers. "God speaks in many and diverse ways to each of us and no one person or one religion has a monopoly on truth."[2] Go directly to Jesus and His word and find yours. You won't find an answer to every question in the Bible, but you will find the character of God; a God who wants to lead you to all you need to know.

Where to start? Perhaps with a bunch of common questions:

*What if God is real?*

*What if the answers to our problems, questions, and fears that exist inside time lie outside time, and therefore, outside our thinking and understanding?*

*What if the conduit to those answers is a God who transcends time?*

*Are there hints of the divine that we have blithely overlooked or obstinately refused to reckon with?*

*Are we marionettes for God's amusement?*

*Are we part of God's human experiment?*

*Are we co-creators participating with a loving God in bringing to completion His kingdom on earth as it is in Heaven?*

## WHERE IS GOD WHEN I NEED HIM? OR HIDE AND SEEK

"There are gifts hidden inside the process of life."[3]

The more I study and ponder the things of God, the more I'm impressed that His mysteries are not hidden, but in plain view right in front of us woven right into our everyday lives. I was playing with my eighteen-month-old granddaughter, Audrey, who was at the bright eyed, bowlegged, waddle, run, stumble, and two syllable stage. Watching her revealed something universal about human behavior. We didn't have to teach her to love cookies and when I first introduced her to a game of hide and seek she got it immediately. I would run off to hide with her baby doll and she would come padding after me, fully engaged in the search.

We all have that aptitude at the get-go and it never leaves. **We are always searching** and hoping to find something. That is what shopping, hunting, and researching are all about. God knows this about us and puts Himself in plain sight, in the beauty of the natural world, the wonder of birth, and the complex order of science. Experience of each other has taught us that we discover something about an artist in his art, and so it is of the Creator in His creation. Unless motivated to search for Him, we never find Him. Cancer, fear, and pain are all great motivators to go searching for Him. He promises that He can be found, but only by those who keep their eyes open and look in His direction.

Now Audrey is three and teaching me something else. She is able to run off and hide on her own and I carry her little sister Ava in my arms while we go look for her. The search no sooner begins than she will make a noise to let us know where she is or jumps out from behind a tree saying, "Here I are." **We all want to be found**; only the children are better at revealing themselves while we adults are better at hiding. The children are the happy ones and we have something to relearn from them about becoming authentic: Here I are God, the real me with all my foibles, fears, and fantasies. Take me as I am and lead me on. He will.

## IS THIS ALL THERE IS? - MONOPOLY

More mysteries are hidden in other games we play. What if our lives were a game within a bigger game, a story within a larger story, an existence within time which extends beyond time? We play board games and sports within the bounds of a playing board or a field, and often within the bounds of a time clock.

We play them with all the gusto and excitement and intrigue of real life and yet they will end and we will move on. We pack the pieces back in the box and the players back on the bus and return to *the rest of our lives.*

The Bible tells us our life is exactly the same. We can live it to the fullest with all the gusto and intrigue of our games, confident that when it is over, there is a hot dinner, warm bed, and family waiting for us, and the rest of *real life* in Heaven. Wouldn't it be easier to live the game of our lives if we were confident that special afterlife in Heaven awaits us. Wouldn't it be easier to, "Go to Jail, Do Not Pass Go, Do Not Collect $200" and Take This Cancer Treatment if you knew that the rest of the real-life was still waiting for you? Wouldn't we enjoy the game of this life more, worry less, and have more fun if we knew that the outcome of the game called *LIFE* wouldn't change the bounty and wonder of the *real life* that lies beyond? My sense is that the only way to arrive at and live in a place of such confidence is to get to know and trust the One who claims it is true and that is Jesus! It is not Buddha, Hare Krishna, the Rising Sun or Mother Earth. That is what a spiritual journey is all about. At least that is where it leads the Windrunners. I have cared for many people who were looking elsewhere, some still looking for the Messiah, but I just never saw any real runners. Walkers some, pretenders a few, and stumblers many, but Windrunners never!

# WHY?

Newton, Einstein, and Edison discovered truths that I would never have discovered and still don't understand very well. However, my limited understanding doesn't in any way lessen their validity. It is so hard to see something that we don't know exists, yet we will never find anything unless we search.

No animal understands the mystery of an image reflected in a mirror. Could they be taught to understand? If God's image is reflected in His creation can we learn to comprehend it? Is it worth a try? Even though we want to know everything about God, is it sufficient to know something? Francis Collins, M.D., PhD, believes that it is. He is a geneticist who led a team of 2000 scientists from six countries In the Human Genome Project which determined all 3 billion letters of the human genome that compose the DNA instruction book for every cell in our bodies. Immersed in scientific inquiry, he began seeing signposts to something outside nature that could only be called God. He realized, "the scientific method can really only answer questions about *how* things work. It can't answer questions about *WHY* – and those are in fact the most important ones. Why is there something instead of nothing? Why does mathematics work so beautifully to describe nature? Why is the universe precisely tuned to make life possible? Why do we humans have a universal sense of right and wrong, and an urge to do the right – even though we may disagree sometimes about what "right" is."[4]

## JIGSAW PUZZLE

The big picture of God is like a jigsaw puzzle. Some of the pieces will come from the Bible, some from other people's experiences, some from our own experiences, some from prayers, and some directly from God. The pieces don't all come in order, but over time a mosaic of the different pieces will form a clearer, more confident picture. Never throw out any piece that doesn't seem to fit, at least not yet, like some peculiarity in another worshiper's life, or something in church history, or an unanswered prayer, or a confusing one. They can all seem disconcerting. Just set them aside. One day as the big picture becomes clearer, there will be a place for those seemingly inconsistent or worthless pieces. Until then, they need not invalidate or spoil your expanding picture. Give them time.

Getting the big picture is more important than understanding every piece. It may seem peculiar that the most important decision of our existence, whether we will surrender our own will to the divine will must be made without complete understanding, but that is where the journey begins and that is the way it is with jigsaw puzzles. You have to start somewhere. You can always stop and throw the puzzle back in the box and you can always take your freewill back.

**Many read the Bible and try to figure out what it means, but Jesus is more direct.**

**He simply invites us to do what He says and discover what it means in the process.**

Even the people who traveled and listened to Jesus for three years back in 29-32 AD didn't understand it all. They stood at the foot of the cross and they didn't get it. They didn't understand the whole notion of Jesus' dying for the sins of mankind in order to make it possible for those who believe in Him to approach God, receive His Spirit, and start experiencing a new dimension of life in relationship with Him. They didn't really get it until they received and start experiencing His Holy Spirit. I still just barely get much of it.

## It's About a Relationship with Jesus, so... Who Is He?

God is the Creator of all things, you and me and everything around us. Only through knowing Him and what He is up to will it all makes sense, hold together, have meaning, and purpose. The creation of His kingdom is the goal. It is ongoing and each of us has an opportunity to contribute and be part of it both now and for all eternity. Who He is has been revealed in His creation, and through His prophets, but is most fully and precisely revealed in the letter He sent to us. That letter was Jesus, the life He lived, the things He did, the things He said, the look in His eyes, and the touch of His hands. Jesus was not just a messenger of God like the prophets, He was and is God speaking a human language, visible to the eye, tangible to the touch, and moving in human history. God moved through the lives of the Jewish people recorded in the Old Testament to set the stage for and point toward the coming of Jesus. It is through the character of Jesus that the fullness of the character of God is revealed. Because words are not enough, Jesus acted out the meaning of the words through His life as recorded in the four Gospels Matthew, Mark, Luke, and John. The overwhelming truth that comes through that record and through the lives of those who know Him, is that He is good and that He loves us. We don't always understand His goodness, particularly at first, but we are all attracted to His unconditional love which is so beyond our human experience. "Every day you wake up, God loves you as you are, not as you should be."[5]

Amid the great recession of the late 2000s that brought so many of us to our knees, Gino Grundberge reminded us, "every setback is a set up for comeback." He introduced Mark Hatteberg who told us some of greatest comebacks of all time: #10 was Elvis when he reinvented himself in 1968 TV special after years of making schlocky movies. #7 was Harry Truman who won the presidency after trailing in the polls by a wide margin. #5 was Muhammad Ali who in 1974, years after being stripped of his title, KO's George Foreman. #3 was Michael Jordan who quits baseball in 1995 to make his first triumphant comeback. #2 are Japan and Germany that rise from the ashes of World War II to become industrial powers the 1950s. #1 is Jesus Christ, 33 A.D.

who defies critics and stuns the Romans with His resurrection. Gino got his point across. Jesus' resurrection is a historical fact. The question is: Are we paying attention and what does it mean?

## CHRISTIANITY – CLIFF NOTES

The Bible tells us that at age thirty-three this man who claimed to be God, surprised His followers by permitting Himself to be crucified, and thereby set the stage for His triumphant, mind-boggling final act: His resurrection. He reappeared in bodily form from the grave having, defeated death once and for all, thereby establishing His divinity and His power, and affirming the kingdom He proclaimed was outside time, beyond the grave, and beyond our comprehension. Skeptics can debate the validity of the historical facts surrounding the empty tomb and Jesus' resurrection. They can question the reliability of the woman who met the resurrected Jesus by the empty tomb or the disciples who shared a breakfast Jesus prepared for them or the hundreds who saw and listened to Him during the forty days He walked the earth after His resurrection. But no one can fail to conclude that something extraordinary happened, something so extraordinary that lives were radically changed and are still being changed. A new hope was born, a hope so powerful that countless people have risked their lives, and many have lost their lives, just to profess it. People don't risk their lives to profess a lie, but most of the twelve disciples were killed for professing the truth of Jesus resurrection, as was the apostle Paul and countless others. Something happened! Something so precious, HOPE came into being and people were willing to pay the ultimate price just to hang onto it. It is the hope of those people who belonged to Jesus then and belong to Jesus now, that they will one day be raised and resurrected just as He was and will be with Him throughout eternity.

To live in the God dimension, in His heavenly kingdom on earth during this life, let alone in Heaven someday, is worth getting to know and bend a knee to Jesus. The hope of resurrection someday with Him has been the adrenaline that powers every Windrunner on their Bell Laps. "The message of Easter is that God's new world has been unveiled in Jesus Christ and that you are now invited to belong to it."[6]

If Jesus were standing before us right now, I think He would be saying, "Ego eimi, I am who I am, the Alpha and the Omega, the Lord God Almighty, and I am alive in Heaven and on earth. Although you can't see Me now, you can see My reflection in the world I created and your friends whose lives I inhabit. Come have a transcendent experience with Me. Let Me unchain your heartstrings so you can vibrate, hear, and feel the wonder of My creation. Experience the majesty of a cathedral and find Me there, a rising tide of prayerful song and find Me there, the tenderness of a friend's love and fellowship and find Me there, the quiet sequestered moments of prayer and meditation and find Me there. I am more real than the chalkboard equations in your mind and every bit as reproducible. Your scientific method requires proofs that can be reproduced by another investigator. Those investigators are all around you and their lives are living publications. They are eager to share what they have learned about Me in the laboratories of their lives. They are just waiting to be asked. So ask! When I return, you will see Me face-to-face and I will make all things new, the earth and heavens and your bodies. I came because I want to connect with you. I want to be in relationship with you and want you to experience with Me the joy and fulfillment of bringing forth My kingdom on earth as it is in Heaven. And I want your help in doing it. PS- Please pay attention."

His message was simple, "I am the bread of life"- you need to feed on Me to sustain the life I've given you. "I am the light of the world" – you need My light to expose the darkness that surrounds you. "I am the good shepherd" I will watch over and protect you. "I am the resurrection and the life" and I have promises for you in this life and beyond. I have a plan for your life which is part of an overall plan far greater than you can know or imagine. You need to trust Me to guide you there. If you do, I will protect you and bring you home with Me to a life eternal, full of health, free from worry, full of fascination without boredom, full of love, and free from fear. It is a place where you will experience the fullness of love and a completeness of purpose (John 6:35, 8:12, 10:11, 11:25).

He has given us enough information to make us curious and enough imagination to tantalize us. He permitted enough traumas to reveal our need for Him. Then He has given us absolute control to decide whether to surrender absolutely that control back to Him. His invitation is daily and lifelong: "Trust Me. Trust Me that I love you. Trust Me that I am good. Trust Me that My plans for you are true and will satisfy your every longing."

Mark Batterson observed in his life, "Sometimes it takes a shipwreck to get us where God wants us to go" (from *Wild Goose Chase*, p. 119). Sometimes our life has to fail in order for His life in us to succeed. Sometimes our agenda has to fail in order for His agenda to succeed. If the life in your body is ebbing out, is it an opportunity for His life in your body to flood in?

## TRUST, WINDRUNNERS' LIFEBLOOD

Trusting God involves submission; they go hand-in-hand. While they can be spoken in an instant, making them a reality is a stepwise process for which we are given a lifetime. In it we discover the fullness of who we are created to be. Indeed, I believe that is the essence of what life is about and why we're here. It won't feel like drudgery or defeat, indeed just the opposite. Every sailor knows what it is like when they are in the groove. When the trim of the sail, the heading of the helm and stability of the keel are in perfect harmony, the vessel finds the sweet spot and surges forward with a speed and grace that is palpable. You can feel it in the seat of your pants and you know the vessel would be singing if it had a voice. Our lives are like that vessel. Whatever the winds may be, whether in storms or doldrums, He will direct life's course to the sweet spot.

## THE REAL JESUS

**Brian McLaren points out there are "many different saviors smuggled in under the name Jesus,** just as many different deities can be disguised under the term God and vastly different ways of living promoted under the name Christianity. Jesus can be the victim of identity theft. People can say and do things in his name that he would never do" - *A New Kind of Christianity* (pg 119). Inspired by the Father of Lies, we remake Jesus in our own image and think of Him as one who loves who we love and hates who we hate, "The white supremacist Jesus, the Republican or Democrat Jesus, the organ music, stained-glass window nostalgic sentimental Jesus, the anti-science know nothing, simpleton Jesus, the male chauvinist Jesus, the anti-Muslim crusader Jesus" (pg 122) or the prosperity Jesus, or the Jesus of our childhood, or the Jesus of the bigots down the street or on the TV. We need to let go of those in order to recognize the real Jesus.

"Hardly anyone who hears the full story of Jesus and learns the true facts of his life and teaching, crucifixion and resurrection, walks away with a shrug of the shoulders, dismissing him as unimportant" (Introduction to Colossians, MSG). To know the real Jesus, you can look to those with eyewitness evidence, the Gospels, and to those with experiential evidence, like Windrunners. Then you should meet Him and decide for yourself.

Another compelling place to start is with the story of a committed atheist and skeptic, Lee Stroebel, who was comfortable believing, "the divinity of Jesus was nothing more than the fanciful invention of superstitious people." Lee Stroebel was a Yale Law School graduate and the legal affairs editor for the Chicago Tribune when he was stunned by wonderful changes in his wife who had become a Christian. Fascinated, he chose to apply the tenacity of investigative journalism and the techniques of legal court room scrutiny to the questions: "Is the Bible a trustworthy record? Is Jesus who He claims to be, the Son of God? Did the resurrection really happen?" He interviewed leading scholars with impeccable academic credentials to explore many avenues of proof, eyewitness evidence, circumstantial evidence, corroborating evidence, rebuttal evidence, documentary evidence, scientific evidence, and even fingerprint evidence. His book that recounts his investigation and personal faith journey, *The Case for Christ* is a compelling read. Another place to go is *Mere Christianity* by an Oxford college professor, C. S. Lewis, another atheist turned Christian apologist.

## GOD'S SCRIPT

*You were given life for a reason and with the purpose, and that hasn't changed with cancer.* Some of the charade you have created for yourself and called your life may be outside God's plan. If so, prudence encourages you to ferret it out and let it go. Otherwise, it will be extra baggage only making your Bell Lap harder. God's patience, love, and forgiveness for you are infinite, but your strength and time are not. God doesn't promise you enough of either strength or time to accomplish both His agenda and yours. You had best stick with His if you really want to get something done and avoid worrying about it.

"God has shaped you for eternal purposes," says Eugene Petersen in *Run With the Horses*. He is the potter, you are the clay, life is the wheel. The pot is never finished until it is molded, glazed, and fired. The time in the furnace is on the Bell Lap when something very important happens. Be alert and open to what God has for you in this time. He isn't done with you yet. It is no time to give up, give in or get distracted; God is at work..

Slowly, something theologians call sanctification or becoming like Christ, happens. Some would say it is about learning to love, forgive, and care for others as Jesus did. Many try on their own without the Holy Spirit and fail because their life and humanity gets in the way. I think Jesus would simply say, "Follow Me. Let My Spirit lead you and the rest will happen.

Learning to open one's heart and mind to follow Jesus takes time and practice and that is why we are given a lifetime to figure it out. It just takes time. It is different from the forgiveness of our sins that leads to redemption and a promise of heaven that comes immediately, completely, and irrevocably for each whom, in contrition bend their knee and invite Christ into their life. So, start cracking your heart open soon.

## NEVER A CONTROLLING GOD

While we may invite God to lead our lives, He never takes control of them. He will never give up on us, but we always have the right to give up on Him. How tender His heart must be to always leave us with such free will to make our own choices while all long hoping that we will choose Him and stick with Him. I love the metaphor which casts the Lord as a Potter (Isaiah 64:8, Jeremiah 18:6) and us as clay. The clay may respond to His forming hands or to unseen natural forces – either gravitational or centripetal. Sometimes the clay behaves as if it has a mind of its own and goes flying off the wheel, but it is never discarded. The Potter just picks it up, roles it up, and starts over again. So it is with our Potter God who doesn't give up on us even when forces of our human nature willfully take us flying off in our own direction. He is always willing to give us another try.

Epicetus, the Greek stoic philosopher, opined, "It is difficulties that show what men are." The corollary is more important: It is the difficulties that are meant to show who God is. "Not a lot is learned in happy snappy land," says Suzy, paraphrasing Gary Thomas' *Sacred Marriage*. "That is why God let there be difficulties in life. They make a perfect arena in which to learn and to get to know Him. He beckons us, 'Come unto Me, all you who are burdened and heavy laden and I will give you rest.'"

We are not a finished product. None of us are. We seldom just transition eagerly from one stage of life to the next easily yielding and surrendering our past life without having it ripped from our grasp. As adults, we lose sight of the fact that we are still becoming and that God is not done with us yet. The backstretch is the perfect time to let Him do His work on us.

You may have run out of ideas, but God hasn't. Just ask Him. He has plans and a purpose for you even on your Bell Lap. He has planned the number of days that He is going to work with you in His earthly workshop and the day is set when He will take you home with Him, either for remedial studies or graduate work. The only question for you now is whether you will let Him finish what He has started. Will you seek His path for you now and run along it, or will you say, "I'm good enough, I know enough, I've seen enough, I've dreamed enough, and now I'm just giving up."

God has written a musical score for your life, set you before a keyboard, and invited you to play. You can bang away like a child and perhaps you may stumble onto a melody, but if you learn to read the music, you'll produce a semblance of melody right away. Practice will perfect it and creativity will produce variations on the theme. This is God's intention. When you live in harmony with His score, you experience the music of heaven in your life - kingdom music. It doesn't take a musician to tell if you are off key or not practicing.

The spirit world is another realm like music. You can't touch or see either one, but you can hear and sense them both. When the music is good, everyone wants to dance. So it is with someone living in harmony with God's intention. Everyone can sense the peace and comfort, and glimpse a piece of heaven. They know there is something special going on and they want to get involved. Sometimes the best evangelism is just ordinary people playing their instruments well and God's kingdom grows.

## THE INCARNATION

God gave the people of Israel the law, in essence saying this is what I need you to be about. This is what's important to Me. When they couldn't follow it, He sent His Son, Jesus, Emmanuel, God with us. God expressed Himself, not just with words but with the life of His Son. Over hundreds of years, His prophets had set the stage so the Israelites were expecting a Messiah.

They expected someone like Moses, a deliverer, or like their King David, a powerful conqueror, or someone who would deliver them from the tyranny of Roman rule by conquering the Roman armies. Many did not recognize Jesus who came with a different kind of power to rescue hearts and lives, bringing deliverance from sin, deceit, bitterness, anger, lust, and greed. Today, we need to do better than the Israelites did 2000 years ago. We need to let Jesus be Jesus and discover who He is rather than looking right past Him expecting something else. That takes an adventure.

We can though expect Him to understand us completely. He understands us not only because He made us, but because He has experienced what is like to be us. Without giving up His deity, He set aside the privileges of deity. In submission to the Father's plan, Christ limited His own power and knowledge and became human, became subject to our limitations of place and time, biology, and psychology, became obedient to fatigue, hunger, thirst, exasperation, anger, affection, and sorrow (Philippians 2:6–8, John 1:1–14, Romans 1:2–5, Hebrews 2:14, I John 1:1–13). He can identify with us in every arena because He has been there. He knew we would feel a kinship for someone who had experienced what we experience.

It is no accident that He had a Bell Lap as well. **Jesus can identify with us in our tribulations and in our desperate prayers when we face life-threatening illness. He prayed them, too.** Clearly there's nothing wrong with such prayer and we need not be timid or ashamed. Fervent prayer is exactly what we are called to and what Christ modeled for us. He also modeled for us an attitude in His prayer, "but please Father, not what I want. What do you want?" (Luke 22:41–44 MSG).

That was a prayer one can only pray if one is totally confident and trusting of the God one prays to. It is a kind of confidence that takes lots of prayer and trust experiments to establish. Notice what happened next, "at once an angel from heaven was at his side strengthening him." That is what we can expect also when we pray from our hearts like that – God's strengthening comfort from the Holy Spirit and sometimes angels, too.

It was no accident that somehow in the mystery of His humanness that coexisted with His godliness, He experienced all the temptations and challenges we now experience. Any human will quickly respond: wait a minute. Jesus never gave in to temptation. He never sinned. That's not me. Not even close. I can't relate!

Consider this. Jesus never said it was easy for Him. Indeed, He got exasperated repeatedly and when the anticipation of torture and death lay before Him, He struggled and prayed for escape with such angst that He sweat blood. We are not meant to understand the intersection of His humanity and His divinity in that moment. We know He prayed some more and remained ever submissive to His Father's will. **Christ did not sidestep temptation, He prevailed over it. He showed us how: He rested on the sufficiency of His Father and the divine plan.** What does that mean?

I think it means all temptation and sin seem to arise from our perception of "not enough" – not enough money, power, acceptance, security, time, life, sex, and ultimately control. I believe that Jesus was able to resist, not because of superhuman divine discipline (although I'm sure He had it), but because of His absolute confidence that in His Father and our God, there

IS ENOUGH of everything; even more and better than we can imagine.

Jesus spent His three-year ministry not touting His willpower and divine power, but describing the sufficiency of God and God's power. The sufficiency that is available to us in this life when we live it in God's dimension, in His kingdom, and in heavenly relationship with Him. The super sufficiency of life beyond death united with Him, in a new body, on a new earth where and when all things are made new and complete. One need not be tempted by another Big Mac, scoop of ice cream or chocolate if one knows that the cupboards at home are always full of them. One doesn't need to scramble for love and self-worth if both are guaranteed, nor power when it has become irrelevant and unnecessary.

The question is ultimately whether such confidence is possible for us, and if so, how do we get it? Until a few years ago I would've said, "That's an interesting question for intellectual debate. Obviously the answer is no, but let's talk about it – preferably over a good beer or at least a good cup of coffee, because it's a rather dry subject for which there can be no definitive answer." Then I started meeting Windrunners. The subject became intriguing and my answer changed.

# THE HOLY SPIRIT –CLIFF NOTES

Old Testament prophets anticipated a time when there would be an outpouring of God's Spirit on His people. Bystanders on the river bank witnessed God's Spirit descend "like a dove" on to Jesus as He rose out of the baptismal waters of the Jordon in the arms of His forerunner nephew John later called the Baptist. They all heard a voice from heaven say, "This is my son, whom I love; with him I am well pleased." After Jesus' resurrection, He appeared to the apostles and He said, "Peace be with you! As the Father has sent me, I am sending you." And with that He breathed on them and said, "Receive the Holy Spirit" (John 20:21). On another occasion when many other believers were gathered, on the day of Pentecost, "Suddenly a sound like the blowing of a violent wind came from heaven and filled the whole house where they were sitting. They saw what seemed to be tongues of fire that separated and came to rest on each of them. All of them were filled with the Holy Spirit" (Acts 2:3).

All throughout Scripture, in both the words of the prophets and Jesus, the Spirit is referred to as the water of life, a metaphor worth pondering. Water is something absolutely essential for life. We become weak, disoriented, incoherent, and die without it. We are restored, energized, coherent, and alive with it. When we drink in Jesus' Spirit that is exactly what happens to our soul. One drink of water is not enough for our bodies. We need to keep returning to the well daily and so it is with Jesus.

When we are cut, bruised, and filthy we are helpless to do anything about it without water to wash away layers of dirt and grime to expose wounds we cannot see and to clean them making healing possible. Jesus' Spirit does that for our souls. Curiously, we seldom think about water until we get thirsty or dirty. That is just what Jesus is waiting for. Are you thirsty yet? The dying usually are. Perhaps a sweet taste of Jesus would be a good idea before your dive in the dirt. Such a simple metaphor, but so powerful and so clever. No wonder Jesus used it so often. "If anyone is thirsty, let him come to me and drink. Whoever believes in me, as the Scripture has said, streams of living water will flow from within him." By this He meant the Spirit (John 7:37-38).

Oswald Chambers points out, "A river is victoriously persistent, it overcomes all barriers." It may encounter an obstacle, but water will keep pouring down from its source and it will surmount the obstacle, going around, over, under or through it. So it is with the rivers of living water, His Spirit, which Jesus pours into us. Rivers are indifferent to an obstacle. They know they will reach the sea. Jesus intends that we be equally confident that our source, Him, will keep pouring Himself into us that we may be confident of our destiny of heaven and indifferent to the obstacles before us. It is not the first splash that overcomes an obstacle, but the continued outpouring that fills us up and breaks through any logjam or carves an entirely new channel. The filling is intended for more than just our immediate need and our own overcoming. "Whoever drinks the water I give him will never thirst. Indeed, the water I give will become in him a spring of water welling up to eternal life" (John 4:14). From this spring will flow living water, the knowledge and experience of Him which is meant to be passed on. (See chapter on Pass the Baton.)

## SENSING THE SPIRIT'S LEADING

Anyone can tell the direction of the wind in a good blow, but sensing the direction of a gentle breeze takes an experienced sailor who can feel a zephyr on his windward cheek and the wind shadow from his nose on his leeward cheek. The mariner can read the wind in the smallest ripple on the face of a calm sea and sense a gathering storm in the character of the clouds. It all takes practice and so does sensing the guiding breath of God's Spirit. It's like a man I saw on a train.

I was fascinated to watch the gentleman pour over the pages of a complex musical score for an orchestra. As I watched, his head and hands would gently bob and weave with music only he could hear. Somehow, he was able to translate the gobbledygook of notes on the page into a musical experience in his head while to me they were only ink spots on the page. I couldn't hear the music. I think God has created notes on a musical score for our lives that we can only understand with the help of the Holy Spirit. Even then they are dry and lifeless notes until we let them play out in the rest of God's story. Then they become real and we experience the music and call it all life and the astonishment begins.

Is it any surprise that God would not limit His truth to the spoken or written word, but instead embodied it in the life and death of His Son and then offers to download it all for free like a smart phone app called GD VISION (God's Dimension Vision -aka the Holy Spirit) into the heart of anyone who is interested. When called up, the Spirit enables connection with God's dimension, sort of like multi-sensory 3-D glasses that are not just for vision but for hearing, feeling, and understanding as well.

If you haven't experienced God's dimension before, you may not recognize it moving through the lives of people all around you. You won't feel the zephyr on your cheek. Even though you might see a ripple on the face of the sea, you won't know what it means. Someone without ears can steadfastly assert there is no such thing as the spoken word or a musical note, let alone a song or a sonata. However, their assertion doesn't make it so. Consider, therefore, could there be a Spirit of God who does speak, and given the chance will create music in your life? Can you imagine the wonder of a deaf man given hearing and awakening to Bach, Santana or Dave Matthews? Could that await you on a cosmic spiritual scale with a JC download?

The Holy Spirit lets you in on "God's secret wisdom" that Paul speaks about in 1 Corinthians 2:9-10, "No eye has seen, no ear has heard, no mind has conceived what God has prepared for those who love him," but God has revealed it to us by His Spirit. The Spirit searches all things, even the deepest things of God and reveals them to those who are paying attention. Some say God doesn't speak today, at least not to them or at least not in any way they can understand. Marcel Marceau and Charlie Chaplin would beg to differ. All they had to say was communicated without words, only with mime, expression, and gesture. God's creation speaks silently with just as much eloquence and you don't have to look far to see He's enjoying Himself. It is for us to let the mystery of God infiltrate our souls and let Him speak specifically to each one of us.

Sometimes His communication is concrete, a word or an idea. Other times it is less so, a notion, a calling, an inspiration or a feeling. Sometimes it's a word from a friend or a pastor or one that leaps off of a page of Scripture. Often He speaks most eloquently to us through the events in our lives in a language only we can understand, but then only if we look back on our lives and reflect. The vocabulary of the Spirit is Scripture. If we haven't read it, we won't recognize the language of the Spirit's whisperings and will limit the Spirit's ability to guide us. The Spirit doesn't invent new truth, He googles or Wikipedia's God's vast library of truth and wisdom and pulls up just what we need at any given moment and displays it on the forefront of our thoughts. If we have read the pertinent scripture before, we will pick up on what the Spirit is trying to say faster. Interpretation can be difficult and that is when wrestling it through with a community of believers becomes so precious.

There are many imperfect voices clamoring to speak into your head, so believers often like to give God a head start first thing as their eyes are opening with a prayer. It's like turning on the radio, finding the right station, and staying tuned in all day. One may periodically need to turn up the volume as the day becomes more hectic. If it is too low or you're on the wrong station, you have eliminated God's ability to help you through.

## IS HE THERE? ARE YOU LISTENING?

If you have never sensed the Spirit's whisper, you have got to be thinking, "What kind of mumbo-jumbo is this guy talking about?" Stay with me here. The Spirit is real, but you can't see it just like you can't see the wind. You only see its effects and when you do, you will know that it is real. The apostle Paul writes in Galatians about the fruit you see in a Spirit filled life, "The fruit of the Spirit is love, joy, peace, patience, kindness, goodness, faithfulness, gentleness and self-control"(5:22). When absent, acts of our sinful human nature prevail: immorality, debauchery, idolatry, hatred, discord, jealousy, fits of rage, selfish ambition, envy, drunkenness, and the like. Every time I recount these lists I recognize another closet in my life into which I need to invite the Holy Spirit, and fortunately a few where it has made real progress. If you have invited Jesus into your life, you can be certain the Spirit is there and just waiting for your attention.

# SELF-DECEPTION

**Self-deception** is common in the Christian community, but there is no time it is more prevalent or its consequences more injurious then when one is faced with a critical illness. People seem to be able to say the most amazing things about their faith without actually believing what they say. It is as if just speaking of faith would give them God's power and protection. But it is only the actions in their lives which reveal what they truly believe in their hearts, and it is that heart belief that gets God's attention. The faith talkers are often disappointed in God and conclude that His plan, power, and protection are a fraud, when it is they who are the fraud and God who will be disappointed. There is no surer road to mediocre Christian living than such an unwitting self-deception.

God cannot do anything with someone who has an uncommitted heart and hiding behind the **charade of words**. They miss out entirely on the adventure and get bored and discouraged. Then when tragedy strikes they find themselves both without God's resources or power. What is worse is that they become a discouragement to all those around them that were fooled by their words.

I am convinced that God lets some things happen in our lives that are clearly beyond our control to compel us to recognize our weaknesses and our need for His help - something He is eager to provide. Not many of us elect to venture beyond our skill sets to take on new challenges in life even when we think God is calling us there. The perception of our own inadequacy stops us cold on the threshold of taking on an endeavor that would require God's intervention for success. Yet, God beckons each of us into exactly such a gambit because that is precisely where we will get to know Him best. Living with cancer may be just such a gambit.

Embarking on a different but equally dangerous adventure with God, Gary Haugen created IJM, International Justice Mission. In *Just Courage*, he recounts how totally impossible the lofty goal of rescuing slaves from Third World brick kilns, sweatshops, and underage brothels was with only the strengths and resources he had or could even imagine. It was entirely clear to him that if this mission, which God had laid on his heart, were to succeed, it would be God's doing. Of course, he needed to show up and seek God's leading and then follow it. To this day he does just that. He shows up, and with his staff, confesses their weakness and inabilities and places their will at God's feet. The success of the mission in the torrid and dangerous back alleys of Southeast Asia and South America is beyond amazing. He says, "I can take my gifts and passions and training and strengths beyond the places of safety and control and into the sphere of the kingdom where I actually need God. Perhaps the first indicator that I am approaching such a place will be seen in my life of prayer."

Mother Teresa had the same attitude. She said that she couldn't imagine doing her work for more than 30 minutes without prayer. If your challenge now is running the Bell Lap and all that it entails in the face of your weakness and uncertainty, are you doing it with prayer every 30 minutes? If not, is it because your Bell Lap is so easy without it or have you given up? If the former, may I suggest you expand your Bell Lap vision until it is clearly beyond yourself in the realm where you need and can experience God. If the latter, be encouraged that you are exactly where God wants to meet you, where He can give you hope and show you His power.

I sincerely believe that the Bell Lap cannot be run well with peace and purpose without God. None of the patients I have known who have run well did it without Him. Recognizing your need for His help to direct your steps and comfort your heart and express His power may be the very reason He has let you come to this place of ultimate vulnerability and weakness.

# BELL LAP WINDRUNNERS &THE DRAGON VANQUISHED

# WORKS CITED

Chapter One - FACING THE BEAR

1    Steve Jobs, Stanford report, June 14, 2005.

Chapter Two – PEACE: THE ESSENCE OF A WINDRUNNER

1    Actress Glenn Close to Robert Redford in the 1984 film *The Natural*.

2    Idleman, Kyle. *Not a Fan*. Grand Rapids, Michigan: Zondervan. 2011.

## Chapter Three – THE TRUST THAT POWERS WINDRUNNERS

1   Wendell Price. president of the Missionary Alliance Seminary (1970s) and pastor of North Seattle Missionary Alliance Church (1980s).


## Chapter Four - LETTING GO, GRABBING HOLD AND HANGING ON

1   Jobs, Steve. Lecture at Stanford. 2xxx.

2   Kirsch, Suzanne. Marriage and Family Therapist. Gig Harbor. 2012.

3   Peterson, Eugene. *Run with the Horses*. Intervarsity Press. Downers Grove, IL. 2009. p. 102.

4   Young, William P. *The Shack*. Windblown Media. Newbury Park, Calif. 2007.

5   Lewis, C.S. *A Grief Observed*. New York. Harper & Row. 1961.

6   Paraphrase from Frederick B. Meyer's book *The Secret of Guidance* as quoted by Dallas Willard. *The Allure of Gentleness*. Pp. 154. 2015. HARPERCOLLINS. NY, NY. 10007.


## Chapter Five – PROFILES IN TRUST

1   Lewis, C.S. *A Grief Observed*. New York. Harper & Row. 1961. p. 34.

2   Furtick, Steven. *Sun Stand Still*.

3   Furtick, Steven. *Sun Stand Still.* p. 12.


Chapter Six – OBSTACLES TO TRUST

1   Manning, Brennan. *Ruthless Trust.* New York, NY: Harper Collins. 2000 quotes Edward Farrel: *Prayer is a Hunger.*

2   Words borrowed from a song by Amy Grant: *Blessings.* 2011.

3   Paraphrased from Kate Bowler. *Death, the Prosperity Gospel and Me.* The New York Times. Feb. 13, 2016.

4   Ibid.


Chapter Seven – CULTIVATING HOPE

1   Paraphrase from *Man's Search for Meaning,* Viktor Frankl, 1946.

2   Lewis, C.S. *A Grief Observed.* New York. Harper & Row. 196.

3   Chesterton, G.K. *Heretics* (London: Bodley Head, 1905), p.114.

4   Georges Bernanos (Philip. Yancey. *Vanishing Grace.* P175. 2014. Zondervan. Grand Rapids, MI.)

5   Petersen, Eugene. *Run with the Horses,* Intervarsity Press, Downers Grove, Il. p. 174.

6   Greenbaum, Norman. *Spirit in the Sky.* Written and Originally recorded 1969.

7   Medved, Michael. *Ten Lies About America.*

8   Jackson, Linda Jo. *I'M FREE*. An excerpt from the poem.

9   Bono, remarks at the President's National Prayer Breakfast 2006.

10  Petersen, Eugene. *Run with the Horses*. Intervarsity Press, Downers Grove, Il. P. 174.

11  Stringfellow, William. *An Ethic for Christians and Other Aliens in a Strange Land*, Waco Tex. Word Bools.1976), p. 52.


Chapter Eight – THE HOPE OF HEAVEN

1   Reeves, Jim. Excerpted from song *This World Is Not My Own*.

2   Rolheiser, Ronald. *The Holy Longing, The Search for Christian Spirituality*. Doubleday, NY. NY. P. 146.

3   Alcorn, Randy. *Heaven*. Tyndale House Publishers. 2004. p. 337.

4   Lewis, C.S.

5   Wright, N.T. *Surprised by Joy*. Harper Collins.

6   Wright, N.T. *Surprised by Joy*. p. 79.

7   Willard, Dallas. The Allure of Gentleness. P68. HarperCollins. NY, NY. 2015

8   Rolheiser, Ronald. *The Holy Longing, The Search for Christian Spirituality*. Doubleday, NY, NY. p. 151.

9   This story has appeared in a variety of forms from which it is paraphrased here. One in particular is *DEADLINE*, Randy Alcorn, Multnomah Books, Sisters, Oregon. P. 65.

10 A line lifted from the movie *The Natural*, Glenn Close speaking to Robert Redford as they reflect on what they are learning form the mistakes in their lives.

11 Knut M. Heim. Psalm 23 in the *Age of the Wolf*. Christianity Today. p. 60. Jan/Feb 2016).

12 CS Lewis. *The Weight of Glory* and other addresses. 1949. MacMillan Publishing Co. NY, NY.

13 CS Lewis. *The Weight of Glory* and other addresses. 1949. MacMillan Publishing Co. NY, NY. p. 12.

14 CS Lewis. *The Weight of Glory* and other addresses. 1949. MacMillan Publishing Co. NY, NY.

15 Donne, John. *Death, Be Not Proud*, The New Oxford Book of English Verse, (Oxford: Oxford University Press, 1972).

16 Schokel, Luis Alonso.

17 Willard, Dallas. *The Allure of Gentleness*. p. 68. HarperCollins. NY, NY. 2015.

Chapter Nine – THE ROAD: PRAYER

1 Paraphrased from Foster, Richard. *Celebration of Discipline: The Path to Spiritual Growth*. Harper Collins. 1978.

2 Sheets, Dutch. *Intercessory Prayer: How God Can Use Your Prayers to Move Heaven and Earth*. Regal. 2008. p. 80.

3   Lane, Robert F. *The Bell Lap. and the Dragon Behind the Door.*

4   Metakis, Eric. Paraphrased from his comments at the National Prayer Breakfast, Washington DC. February, 2012.

5   St. Augustine. Heidelberg Catechism, Q and A 1, OF. per J. Todd Billings. *Rejoicing in Lament.* Brazos Press division of Baker Publishing. 2015. p. 38.

6   Brevard Childs, *Exodus: A Commenty* (London: SCM, 1974), p. 76.

7   Kushner, Harold S. *Conquering Fear.* Random House Inc. 2006 audio book.)

8   Furtick, Steven. *Sun Stand Still.*

9   Brevard Childs, *Exodus: A Commenty* (London: SCM, 1974), p. 22.

10  Brevard Childs, *Exodus: A Commenty* (London: SCM, 1974), p. 23.

Chapter Ten – PRAYER FOR DIVINE HEALING

1   Keefauver, Larry. *When God Doesn't Heal Now.* Thomas Nelson Inc. Nashville, Tenn. 2000.

2   Ibid.

3   Ibid.

Chapter Eleven – A PLACE CALLED PEACE

1   Cappeau de Roquemaure, Placide. *O Holy Night.*

Chapter Twelve – THE BACKSTRETCH

1   Tada, Joni Earekson. www.joniandfriends.org>Radio. May 15, 2013.

2   Unknown

3   Allender, Dan. *TO BE TOLD: God Invites You to Coauthor Your Future.* Waterbrook Press. 2006.

4   Willard, Dallas. *CHOICE IS WHERE SIN DWELLS.*

5   **Building Our Souls**, Rabbi Richard A. Block, Yizkor Sermon, Yom Kippur 5776/2015, Cleveland, Ohio.

6   Kashdan, Todd. Psychology Today July /August 2013. p. 52.

7   Achor, Shawn. *Positivity and Performance. TED Talk.*

8   Heller, Rabbi Zachry I. quoted by Kubler-Ross, Elizabeth. *Death; the Final Stage of Growth.* NY: Simon & Schuster, 1986. P. 40.

9   Piper, Don. *90 MINUTES IN HEAVEN*, Baker publishing group. 2004. p. 20.

10  Lancet 358, number 9298 (December 15, 2001): 2039–45.

11  Levine, Steven. *A Year to Live*, Bell Tower/Crown Publishing, Inc. NYC. 1997.


Chapter Thirteen – PASS THE BATON

1   Hendricks, Howard. *Running to Win.* Worldwide Challenge Magazine, Campus Crusade, Inc. WSN Press, Orlando, Fl. 1989.

2   Peterson, Eugene. *Run with the Horses*. Intervarsity Press. Downers Grove, IL. 2009.

3   The Rolling Stones. *Time is on My Side*. Song lyrics.1964.

4   Chambers, Oswald. *My Utmost for His Highest*. Oswald Chambers. Publication Ltd. 1963.

5   Gladwell, Malcom. *Blink*. Little, Brown and Co. 2005.

6   Coleman, Robert. *The Master Plan of Evangelism*.


Conclusion – THE HOMESTRETCH

1   Karl Barth, *Epistle to the Romans* (London: Oxford University Press, 1960), p. 327.


Appendix 2

1   *Grief Recovery Handbook*, The Grief Recovery Institute 8306 Wilshire Blvd., #21 – a, Los Angeles, CA 90211.

2   Paraphrased from *How to Survive the Loss of Love*, Melba Cosgrove PhD, Harold N. Bloomfield M.D. & Peter McWilliams, 1996, Leo Press, Simon & Shuster.


Appendix 5 – Spiritual Journey

1   Clarke, Chapman. Vice Provost Fuller Seminary. Personal communication 2014.

2    Rolheiser, Ronald. *The Holy Longing*. Doubleday, New York 1999. p. 41.

3   Unknown

4   Collins M.D. Ph.D, Francis S. Presentation at the National Prayer Breakfast, February 1, 2007, Washington, DC.

5   Manning, Brennan. *The Ragamuffin Gospel: Good News for the Bedraggled, Beat-up. and Burned Out.* Multnomah Publishers. Colorado Springs, Co. 2005.

6   Wright, NT. *Surprised by Hope: Rethinking Heaven, the Resurrection and the Mission of the Church.* Harper Collins. p. 253.

# DR. LANE SHARES...

I have been a medical oncologist for over 30 years. Now retired, I can spend time with cancer patients in our community helping them understand what their doctors have said, what their doctors left out and what it all means. Then I help them make decisions that respect their bodies, their families and the life they want to lead.

Early on, I did research on how to control the side effects of cancer chemotherapy and later how to diagnose breast and prostate cancer in the least invasive way then to treat it in a boutique fashion tailored to each patient's unique cancer and circumstances. For years I worked with national cooperative cancer groups: NSABP (National Surgical Adjuvant Breast Project), SWOG (Southwest Oncology Group, and PSOC (Puget Sound Oncology Group) doing clinical research on the characterization and treatment of different cancers. I played a leadership role in conceiving, implementing and then directing a community cancer center, Northwest Cancer Center which evolved into Puget Sound Cancer Centers, then a hospice, Northwest Hospice and later a multidisciplinary breast center, Seattle Breast Center. That center was dedicated to saving breasts and saving lives: both biologic patient lives and their experiential quality. This was achieved through the collaborative efforts of nurses, counselors and clergy and multiple specialty physicians—a practice unheard of then but more common today.

These responsibilities generated an opportunity to speak to patient groups, at conferences and on retreats where the focus has been on both creatively enduring the illness but also prospering and growing through it. I continue to learn from patients and to speak when offered the opportunity.

I presently live on an island in Puget Sound, where I love taking care of the land and the beach when not sailing, climbing, or playing with one with my kids and sibs. I savor fireside reading with my wife and therapist, Suzanne (she is a Marriage and Family Therapist who practices on me regularly). Together we cherish our blended family of nine children and 22 grandchildren. We have started to run our own bell laps without waiting for any disease to ring our bells.

You too can make your bell lap a victory lap. Read my first book, ***CANCER'S BELL LAP and THE DRAGON THE DOOR,*** or check out my blog ***CANCERDOCTALK.COM*** where you can also meet some of the Windrunners and hear their stories in the **BELL LAP DIARIES *(video vignettes)***

*For more resources and connecting with me*
*and my coaching and resources,*
*go to www.cancerdoctalk.com.*

CPSIA information can be obtained
at www.ICGtesting.com
Printed in the USA
BVHW07s1114110618
518747BV00022B/1155/P